WALLABY

THE WILMORE FITNESS PROGRAM

A Personalized Guide to Total Fitness and Health

JACK H. WILMORE, PH.D.

ILLUSTRATIONS BY
Fred Anderson
University of Arizona Health Sciences Center

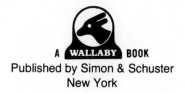

A WALLABY BOOK
Published by Simon & Schuster
New York

WALLABY and colophon are trademarks of Simon & Schuster

First Wallaby Books Printing April 1981
10 9 8 7 6 5 4 3 2 1
Manufactured in the United States of America

Library of Congress Cataloging in Publication Data

Wilmore, Jack H
    The Wilmore fitness program.

    Bibliography: p.
    Includes index.
    1. Physical fitness.   I. Title.
GV481.W564   613.7   80-26770

ISBN 0-671-79143-5

To my wife, Dottie

Acknowledgments

Writing a book involves the efforts of many individuals, most of whom receive little or no recognition. This book would not have been a reality if it weren't for the efforts of the following people. A special thanks to my wife, Dottie, and my daughters, Wendy, Kristy, and Melissa, for their encouragement, and for making sacrifices to allow me time to complete this book; to Mom and Dad for their love and guidance over the years; to my spiritual counselors, the Reverend Ron Ritchie, and Pastors John Dungey and Roger Barrier, for their leadership in helping me establish my priorities as a Christian, and in encouraging my spiritual growth; to all of my professional colleagues who have worked so diligently to establish new frontiers in exercise physiology and sports medicine; and to all of my students, past, present, and future, for providing me with the stimulus to continue to learn and to do my best, and who are a continual source of joy and pleasure.

Special recognition goes to Fred Anderson for the outstanding job he did in providing all of the original illustrations for this book; to Christine Coronado for her conscientious efforts in typing the final manuscript; to Phil Stanforth and Tracy Sullivan for serving as models for many of the photographs used in this book; and to all of the people at Pocket Books and Simon & Schuster who have provided so much help in the final production of this book.

CONTENTS

THE WILMORE FITNESS PROGRAM

A Personalized Guide to Total Fitness and Health

SECTION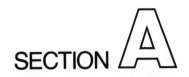

Optimal Health Through Physical Activity and Sport

The beginning of the twentieth century marked a significant period of transition in the history of the United States. Automobiles, airplanes, radios, movies, and the widespread use of the telephone were the more visible symbols of a society which was becoming highly mechanized. As late as the year 1900, 60% of the American population lived on farms or in towns of less than 4,000 inhabitants, and were dependent directly or indirectly on agriculture for their livelihood. With increased mechanization in an age of modern technology, and the general migration of the masses into the cities or urban areas where hard physical labor was replaced by occupations of a highly sedentary nature, man was suddenly confronted with a new life-style which included little, if any, physical activity.

Has man successfully adapted to this change in life-style? The first chapter of this book attempts to answer this question, focusing on those diseases which have been associated with physical inactivity. The second chapter discusses the implications of a more active life-style relative to health and longevity. In short, the initial section of this book describes the health problems associated with our modern life-style, and investigates how increased physical activity through recreational exercises and sport can promote improved health and a sense of well-being.

1

Diseases and Disability Associated with Physical Inactivity

INTRODUCTION

Since the turn of this century, we have witnessed the transformation of a basically hard-working, physically active, rural-based society into a population of anxious and troubled city dwellers and suburbanites who start to sweat and breathe hard at the mere thought of exercise and vigorous physical activity. Heavy, or even moderate, physical activity has become either obsolete or unfashionable. Modern technology has made it possible for us to live comfortably with little expenditure of energy. Hand or push lawnmowers were replaced by power lawnmowers, which, in turn, have been replaced by artificial grass. Elevators and escalators have replaced stairs, making it almost impossible to locate an open stairwell in a modern office building, hotel, or department store. Driving has replaced walking, to the point where anxiety and frustration result from being unable to locate a parking space directly in front of the point of destination—even when there are an abundance of parking spaces within a hundred yards or less walking distance. It is a major family tragedy when the remote control for the television set is suddenly in need of repair. While our bodies are crying out for increased opportunities to be physically active, we are continuously looking for ways to make life even easier, conserving effort and human energy. What do we do with all of this effort and energy that we have saved? Or, possibly, we should ask the question: What does a sedentary life-style do to us as individuals? Do we profit, or do we suffer?

The human body is the most complex entity known to man. Scientists have been attempting to unravel the mysteries of the human body for centuries. While great advances have occurred in gaining an understanding of its basic structure and function, we have only started to scratch the surface. If you have ever taken the time to study the human body and how it works, it is impossible not to be impressed with the delicate and intricate manner in which it functions. The various body systems interact in perfect harmony. One slight disruption to any one part generally affects the body as a whole. Hit the end of your finger with a hammer and notice how the pain shoots up your arm and down the back of your legs to your feet! Or, recall the influence on the total body of a simple cold or headache. We are now beginning to realize that physical inactivity is also a stressor to the body, resulting in major deterioration of normal body function. Such common and serious medical problems as coronary heart disease, hypertension, obesity, anxiety and depression, and lower back problems have been either directly or indirectly associated with a lack of physical activity.

DISEASES ASSOCIATED WITH PHYSICAL INACTIVITY

In 1961, Drs. Hans Kraus and Wilhelm Raab published a book titled *Hypokinetic Disease.** Several years earlier, Dr. Kraus had coined the Greek composite term "hypokinetic"; "hypo" referring to "less than normal," and "kinetic" referring to "active or dynamic." Thus, *hypokinetic diseases* are those diseases which are associated with less than normal activity, or what has been termed physical inactivity.

Coronary Artery Disease

Of the approximately 2,000,000 deaths which occur each year, over 53% of these deaths are the direct result of cardiovascular disease (refer to Figure 1, page 17). The major diseases of the cardiovascular system include high blood pressure and stroke, heart attack, congestive heart failure, rheumatic heart disease, and congenital heart defects. Heart attacks alone accounted for 642,719 deaths in 1975 in the United States, which represented 64.6% of those deaths resulting from cardiovascular disease, or over a third of all deaths during that year! In other words, the summation of all causes of death during that year did not equal the total of those dying from cardiovascular disease; and for every three deaths, one was the result of a heart attack!

Heart attacks are the result of *coronary artery disease,* or *atherosclerosis* of the *coronary arteries.* The coronary arteries are those arteries which supply the *myocardium* or heart muscle with blood and nutrients, and remove waste products. Atherosclerosis is a slow progres-

---

*Kraus, H. and W. Raab. *Hypokinetic Disease.* Springfield, Illinois: Charles C Thomas, Publishers, 1961.

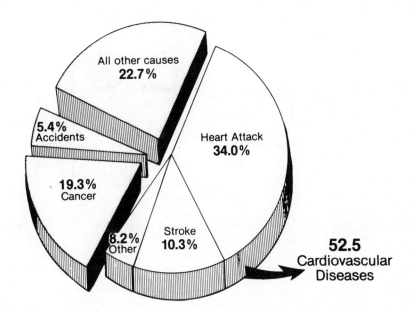

FIGURE 1. Leading causes of death in the United States in the 1970s

sive disease, where the linings of the arteries become thickened and roughened by deposits of fat, *fibrin,* cellular debris, and calcium. Figure 2 (page 18) illustrates the progressive nature of this disease. As the lining of the coronary artery becomes more thickened, the area through which the blood can flow is narrowed, making it difficult to meet the demands of the heart when it is under stress, such as during exercise. Also, if a clot forms in this area, or if a clot forms in another region and breaks lose and lodges in this narrowed channel, the artery becomes blocked, depriving the heart muscle which it supplies of the necessary nutrients and oxygen. It is this blockage of a coronary artery which precipitates a heart attack, and that portion of the heart muscle which was supplied by that artery beyond the blockage dies (see Figure 3, page 18). The greater the area supplied by that artery, the larger the area of heart muscle that dies, and the more severe the resulting heart attack. The left coronary artery, which supplies the left side of the heart, and most importantly the *left ventricle,* is particularly vulnerable. The left ventricle is that part of the heart which must pump blood through the arterial system, throughout the entire body. Extensive damage to the muscular wall of the left ventricle is quite serious, and frequently results in death. A heart attack is also referred to as a *myocardial infarction* (M.I.), *coronary thrombosis* (thrombus is a blood clot), or *coronary occlusion.*

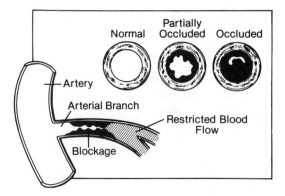

FIGURE 2. The progressive narrowing of a coronary artery, from a cross-sectional view

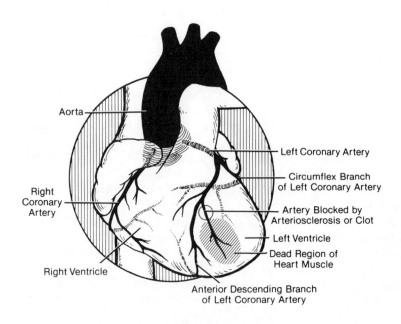

FIGURE 3. Diagram of the heart and its blood supply through the coronary arteries. Notice the small branch off of the anterior descending branch of the left coronary artery. It has become occluded, resulting in a heart attack, and death of the tissue supplied by that branch.

The narrowing of the coronary arteries is a long and slow process that appears to have its origins early in life. Kannel and Dawber, writing in the *Journal of Pediatrics* in 1972, stated that atherosclerosis is not only a disease of the aged, but is primarily a pediatric problem. They cite evidence to indicate that the pathological changes which lead to atherosclerosis begin in infancy and progress during childhood. A study of Korean War combat casualties, with an average age of 22.1 years, revealed that 77% of these young men had at least moderately advanced coronary atherosclerosis. A more recent study demonstrated evidence of atherosclerosis in 45% of a group of Vietnam War combat casualties, with 5% exhibiting severe coronary atherosclerosis.

The natural history of atherosclerosis can be divided into three stages: (1) an incubation period which starts early in life and continues throughout adolescence; (2) a latent period which is asymptomatic, *i.e.,* without symptoms, but in which definite pathological changes can be demonstrated at an early age; and (3) a clinical period during which signs and symptoms first appear. The incubation period is characterized by fatty streaks in the arterial wall. This is the earliest gross pathological alteration that can be seen. By the age of three years, fatty streaks are present in the *aorta, i.e.,* the large artery through which the blood leaves the left ventricle of the heart, of almost all children regardless of their geographical location or diet. During the latent period, beginning in the second decade, the fatty streaks increase in number, size, and distribution, and first become evident in the coronary arteries. The fatty streak is considered to be reversible with changes in diet and exercise habits, among others. If there is no intervention with the progression of the fatty streak, the most commonly accepted hypothesis suggests that the fatty streak progresses to a *fibrous plaque* during the third decade of life. This stage of development is considered irreversible. The clinical period of the disease is that period in which the fibrous plaque has progressed to the point where there is significant narrowing of the coronary artery, sufficient to prevent the heart from receiving the blood it needs during periods of stress.

When the blood flow to the heart muscle is inadequate to meet its needs, as a result of the narrowed coronary arteries, that part of the heart muscle becomes *ischemic* (local and temporary deficiency of blood), and this is referred to as *myocardial ischemia*. Most individuals who have episodes of myocardial ischemia, usually associated with exertion, have extreme chest discomfort or pain, referred to as *angina pectoris*. Often, the pain radiates down the left shoulder and arm, and is usually moderate to extreme in intensity. There is a large percentage of the population, however, which has the same degree of myocardial ischemia, but no associated pain. Approximately 5% to 10% of the "normal" population fall into this category, and they have what is commonly referred to as *"silent heart disease."*

There is still considerable debate as to the etiology or cause of coronary artery disease. Many research investigations have been conducted using both animal and human models, yet the disease process remains largely a mystery. There have been many approaches taken in the study of coronary artery disease, but one of the more interesting and productive approaches, with possible immediate implications, has been the epidemiologic approach. *Epidemiology* is that field of science which studies relationships of those various factors which determine the frequencies and distributions of a particular infectious disease, process, or physiological state. With respect to coronary artery disease, entire communities or populations have been studied for long periods of time, up to several decades in length. Usually included in this type of study are annual or biannual medical examinations, in addition to a comprehensive family and personal medical history.

As an example of this approach, in 1949, the National Heart Institute, now the National Heart, Lung, and Blood Institute, began a prospective epidemiological investigation of coronary artery disease in Framingham, Massachusetts, which has become known as the "Framingham Study." Although federal funding of the long-term study was terminated in the early 1970s, the community has continued to support the costs associated with conducting the project, although at a reduced level, to allow continuation of the project. Over a period of years, many individuals in the community being studied die from a variety of causes, but a substantial number from coronary artery disease. By reviewing the medical histories of those who die from coronary artery disease, is it possible to see what medical abnormalities or problems these individuals have in common. From the Framingham Study, and from epidemiological studies conducted in other communities, a consistent pattern has evolved. A number of factors have been identified, which, when present, place the individual at an increased risk for coronary artery disease. These factors include the following:

Factors That Cannot Be Altered

- heredity
- sex
- race
- age

Factors That Can Be Altered

Primary
- cigarette smoking and possibly other tobacco use

- hypertension or high blood pressure
- elevated serum cholesterol, triglycerides, or low density lipoproteins

Secondary
- diet
- physical inactivity
- obesity
- diabetes
- emotional stress and anxiety
- electrocardiogram abnormalities

Of those factors which can be altered, three are considered to be of significantly greater importance, and are referred to as primary risk factors. Cigarette smoking, *hypertension* or high blood pressure, and elevated blood fats are considered by most researchers and clinicians to be the most critical or important risk factors. Figure 4 (below) illustrates the influence of the presence of one or more of the primary risk factors on

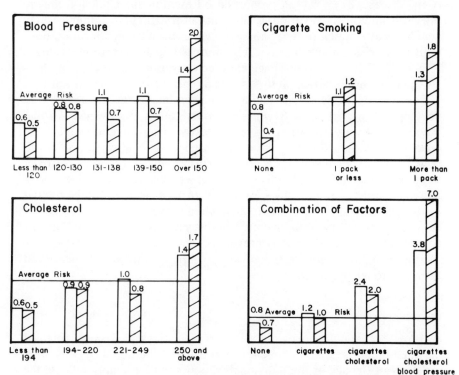

FIGURE 4. Increased risk of heart attack (open columns) and stroke (hatched columns) with one or more of the primary risk factors (Data is from the Framingham, Massachusetts, Heart Study)

the increasing risk for heart attack or stroke. It is important to note that the individual who has all three primary risk factors is at 5.0 times greater risk for heart attack, and 10.6 times greater risk for stroke than the individual who has none of these three risk factors. It is tempting to postulate that the individual who stops smoking and reduces his *cholesterol* and blood pressure to normal levels will decrease his or her risk for heart attack and stroke to the level of the individual with no risk factors, but evidence is incomplete at this time. The American Heart Association has stated that it believes that risk factor modification will reduce the risk for heart attack and stroke to the level of the individual with no risk factors, and that the greatest improvement will result from the simultaneous reduction of all possible factors. Since research has already demonstrated marked coronary artery disease in young men, it is obvious that a 40- or 50-year-old man who smokes two packs of cigarettes a day, has high blood pressure, and has elevated levels of cholesterol will already have significant narrowing of the coronary arteries. However, it is hoped that altering risk factors by changing one's life-style will alter the course of the disease, or its rate of progression. Research and clinical trials are presently under way in various communities throughout the United States which are attempting to determine whether risk factor modification does reduce the risk for the disease. The Multiple Risk Factor Intervention Trial (M.R.F.I.T.) study is specifically investigating the efficacy of altering the three primary risk factors.

The American Heart Association has also made the statement that developing a pattern in early childhood which tends to prevent controllable risk factors from developing is the best way to prevent or delay the onset of heart attack and stroke in later years. It would seem prudent to recommend avoidance of tobacco, control of blood pressure, control of body weight to a desirable level, eating a well-balanced diet with foods low in saturated fat and cholesterol, regular daily exercise, and a regular medical examination starting at a very early age. While there is not sufficient "hard" or irrefutable evidence to prove beyond doubt that this course of action will absolutely prevent coronary artery disease, there is a wealth of indirect evidence that would indicate this to be the sound approach to leading a healthy life.

Hypertension

Hypertension is the medical term used to signify a persistently high or elevated blood pressure, above levels considered normal or desirable on the basis of the age of the individual. Blood pressure simply reflects the pressure exerted by the blood on the vessels through which it flows, similar to the way water pressure reflects the pressure of water on the pipes through which it flows. Water pressure is typically constant, *i.e.,* you open the faucet and water runs out at a rate dictated by the existing water pressure. Blood pressure does not remain constant, but changes with each beat of the heart. As the heart contracts, it pumps blood out of the heart and into the arteries, thus increasing the pressure within the arteries. This peak pressure, which follows each contraction of the heart, is referred to as the *systolic blood pressure*. As the heart relaxes, preparing for the next contraction, the blood pressure within the artery drops to its lowest level, which is referred to as the *diastolic blood pressure*. A *sphygmomanometer* is an instrument used to measure blood pressure, and includes an air-inflatable cuff which is placed around the arm just above the elbow, and a gauge or mercury column from which the blood pressure readings are taken. A *stethoscope* is a device that amplifies the sounds of the blood as it flows through the artery. When the sphygmomanometer is placed on the upper arm and inflated to a pressure above that of the systolic pressure, the underlying artery collapses, and blood flow ceases and no sounds are heard. As the pressure in the cuff is reduced, the sounds will return at that point where the systolic pressure is equal to or slightly greater than the pressure in the cuff, indicating blood is again flowing through that artery. When the cuff pressure drops below the diastolic pressure, the sound will disappear once again, although a change in sound will occur just prior to the disappearance of sound, and this is typically recorded as the diastolic pressure.

High blood pressure is recognized as a silent, mysterious disease, which kills many thousands of Americans each year. It has no specific warning symptoms, thus millions of Americans have the disease, but have no indication that it is present. The cause of hypertension is unknown in more than 90% of those individuals found to be hypertensive, and there is no cure for this disease. Recent research has demonstrated, however, that altered diet, weight reduction, and increased exercise can reduce abnormally elevated blood pressure to normal or near-normal levels. A study reported in 1978 in the *New England Journal of Medicine* found that weight reduction alone had a substantial influence on the reduction of blood pressure in those that were hypertensive. Of 57 patients, all but two showed meaningful reductions in blood pressure, and 61% returned to normal blood pressure values. Medication has also been found to be effective in treating hypertension, but, again, hypertension can only be controlled, not cured, so medication would have to be continued indefinitely.

Recent estimates suggest that 13% of the white male, 25% of the black male, 17% of the white female, and 28% of the black female adult population, age 20 years and above, have hypertensive disease. In the year 1975, it was estimated that over 24,000,000 Americans had hypertension, but as many as 30% of these, or more, were unaware that they had the disease. What is considered to be abnormally high blood pressure?

Most clinicians would agree that a systolic blood pressure in excess of 140 to 150 millimeters of mercury, and/or a diastolic pressure in excess of 110 to 120 millimeters of mercury would be levels of concern in adults. Levels of concern would be substantially less in children. Periodic blood pressure checks are a very inexpensive form of preventive medicine. It takes only a few minutes of time, and could save a life!

Obesity

It has been stated that obesity is this country's "gross national product." It is true that obesity has become a problem of epidemic proportions in the United States. What a paradox—that while people in many parts of this world are starving to death, we are literally eating ourselves to death! Unfortunately, it is difficult to determine just how many Americans are obese, since *obesity* is defined as being overfat. *Overweight* is defined as exceeding the maximum weight listed by sex, height, and frame size in a table of standard values. Unfortunately, the standard tables represent only average or normative data for the population as a whole, and don't take into consideration the composition of the body. There are many individuals who are overweight on the basis of the standard height-weight tables, yet who have a normal or lower than normal amount of body fat. Thus, they are overweight, yet not obese (overfat). Many athletes tend to fall into this category as a result of their heavy bones and large muscle mass. Others fall within the prescribed range of weights for their heights and frame size, yet have more than a normal amount of body fat. They would be obese, yet of "normal" weight. Thus, we should concern ourselves with evaluating the degree of obesity of each individual, and not be overly concerned with whether that individual is overweight, underweight, or of normal weight. As an example, in a study we conducted of 180 professional football players, these athletes had an average height of 6 feet, 2 inches, and an average weight of 220 pounds. According to the standard height-weight tables, these athletes should have had an average weight of not more than 194 pounds. Therefore, they were 26 pounds overweight! When we assessed their body composition by techniques to be described later, we found them to have an average of only 13.5% body fat, which is considerably below the average for their age. They were overweight, yet underfat!

How are overweight and obesity assessed? As was mentioned above, overweight simply implies that the individual exceeds a range of weights specified by sex, height, and frame size. The Metropolitan Life Insurance Company of New York developed tables of desirable weights for men and women in the year 1960. Their data was taken from the 1959 Build and Blood Pressure study of the Society of Actuaries. These tables are reproduced in Table 1 (page 25), and are intended to be used only for those individuals 25 years of age or older. Desirable weight tables are

TABLE 1. Desirable weights for men and women, 25 years of age and over; from the Metropolitan Life Insurance Company of New York, 1960

MEN

HEIGHT		SMALL FRAME	MEDIUM FRAME	LARGE FRAME
Feet	Inches			
5	2	112-120	118-129	126-141
5	3	115-123	121-133	129-144
5	4	118-126	124-136	132-148
5	5	121-129	127-139	135-152
5	6	124-133	130-143	138-156
5	7	128-137	134-147	142-161
5	8	132-141	138-152	147-166
5	9	136-145	142-156	151-170
5	10	140-150	146-160	155-174
5	11	144-154	150-165	159-179
6	0	148-158	154-170	164-184
6	1	152-162	158-175	168-189
6	2	156-167	162-180	173-194
6	3	160-171	167-185	178-199
6	4	164-175	172-190	182-204

WOMEN

HEIGHT		SMALL FRAME	MEDIUM FRAME	LARGE FRAME
Feet	Inches			
4	10	92- 98	96-107	104-119
4	11	94-101	98-110	106-122
5	0	96-104	101-113	109-125
5	1	99-107	104-116	112-128
5	2	102-110	107-119	115-131
5	3	105-113	110-122	118-134
5	4	108-116	113-126	121-138
5	5	111-119	116-130	125-142
5	6	114-123	120-135	129-146
5	7	118-127	124-139	133-150
5	8	122-131	128-143	137-154
5	9	126-135	132-147	141-158
5	10	130-140	136-151	145-163
5	11	134-144	140-155	149-168
6	0	138-148	144-159	153-173

based on the concept that once growth in height stops, there is no biological need for further gains in weight, excluding periods of pregnancy. The weights in these tables were obtained with the individuals wearing shoes and indoor clothing. To translate these figures to nude weights without shoes, you should add one inch for heels in men and two inches for heels in women, and subtract five to seven pounds for clothing.

However, the allowance for shoes is almost equally balanced by the allowance for indoor clothing, so the tables can be used directly, *i.e.,* with your actual height in bare feet and your nude weight, with little or no loss in accuracy.

When using tables such as these to determine desirable weights, it is necessary to know your frame size. How does one determine his or her frame size? Unfortunately, when these tables were originally developed, there was no indication given as to how to estimate frame size. Subsequent attempts have met with little success. It can only be assumed that those with thick chests, broad shoulders, broad hips, and large or thick wrists are to be considered as large-framed, and those with thin chests, narrow shoulders, narrow hips, and small or thin wrists are considered small-framed, with those in between to be considered as medium-framed. Unfortunately, too many individuals use frame size to justify their present weight. It is interesting to note that while bone size remains stable once one reaches maturity, the frame size tends to increase from small to medium, and then medium to large, in direct proportion to one's increase in body weight over the years!

How accurate are these tables for determining one's ideal or desirable weight? If you happen to fall directly at the midpoint of the population for your height, the tables will be adequate. Unfortunately, few people represent the average for the population, thus the tables can be in error for a substantial percentage of the total population. The previous example of the professional football players is obvious, since football players are necessarily heavily muscled and large boned in order to survive the violent nature of the game. However, there is a moderately high percentage of the total population that are labeled overweight, but because of a disproportionately high amount of muscle and bone, they have normal or below normal levels of fat. An equal percentage of the population fall to the other extreme, *i.e.,* they are considered to be of normal or desirable weight by the standard tables, but have an excessive amount of body fat and a disproportionately low amount of muscle and bone. The standard tables only allow you to compare your weight against the normal values for that segment of the male or female adult population that has the same height and frame size. Considering the inaccuracies of these tables on the basis of their inability to differentiate the composition of the body, *i.e.,* bone, muscle, and fat, and the fact that for any one category of height and frame size the weights will range from 7 to 24 pounds, one must conclude that the standard tables for determining desirable weight are of little if any value in helping the individual determine his or her best or ideal body weight.

What are the alternatives, if any? The actual amount of fat weight and *lean body weight* tissue (muscle, bone, organs, skin, etc.) can be determined in the laboratory through various scientific techniques. The most widely used technique, and possibly the most accurate technique, is the *hydrostatic weighing* technique, where the individual is weighed while totally submerged underwater. The weight is taken at that point when the individual has exhaled all of the air out of the lungs (Figure 5, below). This weight is then corrected for the buoyancy effect of additional air trapped in the lungs and pockets of gas in the stomach and intestines. Archimedes discovered several thousand years ago that the volume of an object can be determined by its loss of weight in water, *i.e.,* actual weight − weight underwater. Knowing the volume of a body and its mass or weight, it is possible to calculate the density of that body, since density = mass ÷ volume.

How does the above relate to body composition? The density of pure fat is known, and is substantially less than the density of water, thus fat will float on water. The density of the lean tissue (muscle, bone, organs, skin, etc.) has been estimated, and is substantially above that of water. In simple terms, an obese individual with a large amount of body fat will have a low body density, and will float with ease when placed into a swimming pool. The lean individual with small amounts of body fat will

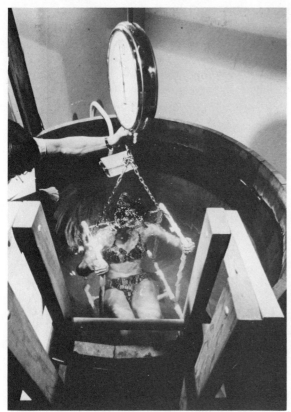

FIGURE 5.

The hydrostatic weighing technique, to determine body composition

have a high body density, and will find it nearly impossible to float when placed into that same swimming pool. As a second illustration, taking two men of exactly the same height and weight, but one is very fat and the other is very lean, the fat individual will weigh much less than the lean individual when weighed underwater, even though their actual weights are identical.

From body density, equations have been established over the years which allow the estimation of *relative body fat,* or that percentage of the total body weight which is fat. As an example, an individual who weighed 200 pounds and was determined to be 20% body fat would have 40 pounds of fat (200 pounds x's 20%) and 160 pounds of lean tissue (200 pounds − 40 pounds of fat). Is 20% too high, too low, or just right? The answer to this question depends only on your sex. Men should be between 12% and 17% body fat, while women should be between 19% and 24% body fat. Any value in excess of 25% body fat for men and 30% body fat for women would be considered obese, and any value in between 20% to 25% for men and 25% to 30% for women would be considered borderline obesity. To determine the ideal or desirable body weight for an individual, you simply divide the individual's lean body weight by that fraction of his or her weight that you want to be lean.

The following example should provide a summary of everything discussed above. Mr. Jones and Mr. Smith come to the University of Arizona to have their ideal body weight determined. By weighing them underwater, the following values were obtained, assuming that 15% body fat or 85% lean body weight is the desired body composition.

	Mr. Jones		Mr. Smith	
Age, years	45		42	
Height	70.0 in.	177.8 cm.	70.0 in.	177.8 cm.
Weight	195 lb.	88.4 kg.	195 lb.	88.4 kg.
Underwater Weight		5.5 kg.		2.5 kg.
Volume (Weight–Underwater Weight)		82.9 kg.		85.9 kg.
Density (Mass or Weight/Volume)		1.066 gm/ml		1.029 gm/ml
Relative Fat		14.2%		31.0%
Fat Weight (Relative Fat x's Weight)	27.7 lb.	12.6 kg.	60.4 lb.	27.4 kg.
Lean Body Weight (Total Weight − Fat Weight)	167.3 lb.	75.8 kg.	134.6 lb.	61.0 kg.
Ideal Weight (Lean Body Weight/0.85*)	197 lb.	89.2 kg.	158.3 lb.	71.8 kg.
Weight Loss (Total Weight − Ideal Weight)	none	none	37 lb.	16.6 kg.

---

*0.85 is the fractional equivalent of 85%, which represents the stated desired fraction of the total body weight constituted by the lean body weight.

From this example, it is obvious that Mr. Jones is heavily muscled and probably large boned, while Mr. Smith is obese. While they weigh the same at the present time, Mr. Jones is already below his projected weight for 15% body fat, while Mr. Smith will have to lose 37 pounds to get to his desirable weight of 158 pounds. According to Table 1, both men are equally overweight by a minimum of 21 pounds if they were considered to be of large frame. The relative body fat values for male and female athletes in various sports are presented in Table 2 (below), to illustrate the wide range of values in a group of individuals who are considered to be in optimal health.

TABLE 2. Body composition values in male and female athletes

ATHLETIC GROUP OR SPORT	RELATIVE BODY FAT, %	
	MALES	FEMALES
Baseball	10–15	–
Basketball	7–12	18–27
Canoeing	10–14	–
Football	8–18	–
Gymnastics	3–6	8–18
Ice Hockey	12–16	–
Jockeys	6–16	–
Skiing		
Alpine	10–17	–
Cross-Country	7–13	18–24
Nordic	8–14	–
Ski-Jumping	12–16	–
Soccer	7–12	–
Speed-Skating	8–14	–
Swimming	4–10	12–20
Track and Field		
Runners	4–12	8–18
Jumpers/Hurdlers	–	12–22
Discus	12–18	22–28
Shot Put	14–20	23–30
Tennis	12–16	–
Volleyball	–	20–23
Weightlifting	6–16	–
Wrestling	6–12	–

Obviously, it would be impossible to weigh the entire population of the United States underwater to determine actual body fat levels, so what are the alternatives? Over the past several decades, scientists have been experimenting with various techniques which would allow an estimation of body fat from one or several easily obtainable measurements. The most accurate of these techniques uses a skinfold caliper to measure the thickness of two layers of skin and the layer of fat which is interposed between the layers of skin. Measurements are taken at six different sites and the resulting values are summed and are used to estimate relative body fat through a series of equations, which have been simplified into several tables for convenience of use. Tables 3, 4, and 5 (pages 30-32) provide estimates of relative body fat from the sum of six skinfolds. Figures 6 through 11 (pages 33-34) illustrate the technique for obtaining accurate skinfold measurements at the specific sites.

TABLE 3. Relative body fat from the sum of six skinfolds in adult women

SUM OF 6 SKINFOLDS	AGE TO LAST YEAR								
	18 to 22	23 to 27	28 to 32	33 to 37	38 to 42	43 to 47	48 to 52	53 to 57	58 and older
38– 42	11.0	11.2	11.3	11.5	11.6	11.8	11.9	12.1	12.2
43– 47	12.3	12.4	12.6	12.7	12.9	13.0	13.2	13.3	13.5
48– 52	13.5	13.7	13.8	14.0	14.1	14.3	14.4	14.6	14.7
53– 57	14.7	14.9	15.0	15.2	15.3	15.5	15.6	15.8	15.9
58– 62	15.9	16.1	16.2	16.4	16.5	16.7	16.8	17.0	17.1
63– 67	17.1	17.2	17.4	17.5	17.7	17.8	18.0	18.1	18.3
68– 72	18.2	18.3	18.5	18.6	18.8	19.0	19.1	19.3	19.4
73– 77	19.3	19.4	19.6	19.7	19.9	20.1	20.2	20.4	20.5
78– 82	20.4	20.5	20.7	20.8	21.0	21.1	21.2	21.4	21.6
83– 87	21.4	21.6	21.7	21.9	22.0	22.2	22.3	22.5	22.6
88– 92	22.4	22.6	22.7	22.9	23.0	23.2	23.4	23.5	23.7
93– 97	23.4	23.6	23.7	23.9	24.0	24.2	24.3	24.5	24.7
98–102	24.4	24.6	24.7	24.9	25.0	25.2	25.3	25.5	25.6
103–107	25.4	25.5	25.7	25.8	26.0	26.1	26.3	26.4	26.6
108–112	26.3	26.4	26.6	26.7	26.8	27.0	27.2	27.3	27.5
113–117	27.2	27.3	27.5	27.6	27.8	27.9	28.1	28.2	28.4
118–122	28.0	28.2	28.3	28.5	28.6	28.8	28.9	29.1	29.2
123–127	28.9	29.0	29.2	29.3	29.5	29.6	29.8	29.9	30.1
128–132	29.7	29.8	30.0	30.1	30.3	30.4	30.6	30.7	30.8
133–137	30.5	30.6	30.8	30.9	31.1	31.2	31.4	31.5	31.7
138–142	31.2	31.4	31.5	31.7	31.8	32.0	32.1	32.3	32.4
143–147	31.9	32.1	32.2	32.4	32.6	32.7	32.8	33.0	33.2
148–152	32.6	32.8	33.0	33.1	33.3	33.4	33.6	33.7	33.9
153–157	33.3	33.5	33.6	33.8	33.9	34.1	34.2	34.4	34.5
158–162	34.0	34.1	34.3	34.4	34.6	34.7	34.8	35.0	35.2
163–167	34.6	34.8	34.9	35.1	35.2	35.4	35.5	35.7	35.8
168–172	35.2	35.4	35.5	35.7	35.8	36.0	36.1	36.3	36.4
173–177	35.8	35.9	36.1	36.2	36.4	36.5	36.7	36.8	37.0
178–182	36.3	36.5	36.6	36.8	36.9	37.1	37.2	37.4	37.5
183–187	36.8	37.0	37.1	37.3	37.4	37.6	37.8	37.9	38.1
188–192	37.3	37.5	37.6	37.8	37.9	38.1	38.2	38.4	38.5
193–197	37.8	38.0	38.1	38.3	38.4	38.6	38.7	38.9	39.0
198–202	38.2	38.4	38.5	38.7	38.8	39.0	39.1	39.3	39.5
203–207	38.7	38.8	39.0	39.1	39.3	39.4	39.6	39.7	39.9
208–212	39.0	39.2	39.3	39.5	39.6	39.8	40.0	40.1	40.3

Sum of chest, thigh, suprailium, abdomen, triceps, and subscapula skinfolds

From M. L. Pollock and A. S. Jackson with permission (personal communication)

TABLE 4. Relative body fat from the sum of six skinfolds in adult men under 40 years of age

Sum of chest, thigh, suprailium, abdomen, triceps, and subscapula skinfolds

				AGE TO LAST YEAR				
Sum of 6 Skinfolds	Under 19	20 to 22	23 to 25	26 to 28	29 to 31	32 to 34	35 to 37	38 to 40
17– 23	.9	1.3	1.7	2.1	2.5	2.9	3.3	3.7
24– 30	2.3	2.7	3.1	3.5	3.9	4.3	4.7	5.1
31– 37	3.7	4.1	4.5	4.9	5.3	5.7	6.1	6.5
38– 44	5.1	5.5	5.9	6.3	6.7	7.1	7.5	7.9
45– 51	6.4	6.8	7.2	7.6	8.0	8.4	8.8	9.2
52– 58	7.7	8.1	8.5	8.9	9.3	9.7	10.1	10.5
59– 65	9.0	9.4	9.8	10.2	10.6	11.0	11.4	11.8
66– 72	10.2	10.6	11.0	11.4	11.8	12.2	12.6	13.0
73– 79	11.5	11.9	12.3	12.7	13.1	13.5	13.9	14.3
80– 86	12.7	13.1	13.5	13.9	14.3	14.7	15.1	15.5
87– 93	13.8	14.2	14.6	15.0	15.4	15.8	16.2	16.6
94–100	15.0	15.4	15.8	16.2	16.6	17.0	17.4	17.8
101–107	16.1	16.5	16.9	17.3	17.7	18.1	18.5	18.9
108–114	17.1	17.5	17.9	18.3	18.7	19.1	19.5	19.9
115–121	18.2	18.6	19.0	19.4	19.8	20.2	20.6	21.0
122–128	19.2	19.6	20.0	20.4	20.8	21.2	21.6	22.0
129–135	20.2	20.6	21.0	21.4	21.8	22.2	22.6	23.0
136–142	21.2	21.6	22.0	22.4	22.8	23.2	23.6	24.0
143–149	22.1	22.5	22.9	23.3	23.7	24.1	24.5	24.9
150–156	23.0	23.4	23.8	24.2	24.6	25.0	25.4	25.8
157–163	23.9	24.3	24.7	25.1	25.5	25.9	26.3	26.7
164–170	24.8	25.2	25.6	26.0	26.4	26.8	27.2	27.6
171–177	25.6	26.0	26.4	26.8	27.2	27.6	28.0	28.4
178–184	26.4	26.8	27.2	27.6	28.0	28.4	28.8	29.2
185–191	27.1	27.5	27.9	28.3	28.7	29.1	29.5	29.9
192–198	27.9	28.3	28.7	29.1	29.5	29.9	30.3	30.7
199–205	28.6	29.0	29.4	29.8	30.2	30.6	31.0	31.4
206–212	29.3	29.7	30.1	30.5	30.9	31.3	31.7	32.1
213–219	29.9	30.3	30.7	31.1	31.5	31.9	32.3	32.7
220–226	30.6	31.0	31.4	31.8	32.2	32.6	33.0	33.4
227–233	31.2	31.6	32.0	32.4	32.8	33.2	33.6	34.0
234–240	31.7	32.1	32.5	32.9	33.3	33.7	34.1	34.5
241–247	32.3	32.7	33.1	33.5	33.9	34.3	34.7	35.1
248–254	32.8	33.2	33.6	34.0	34.4	34.8	35.2	35.6
255–261	33.3	33.7	34.1	34.5	34.9	35.3	35.7	36.1
262–268	33.7	34.1	34.5	34.9	35.3	35.7	36.1	36.5
269–275	34.1	34.5	34.9	35.3	35.7	36.1	36.5	36.9
276–282	34.5	34.9	35.3	35.7	36.1	36.5	36.9	37.3
283–289	34.9	35.3	35.7	36.1	36.5	36.9	37.3	37.7
290–296	35.2	35.6	36.0	36.4	36.8	37.2	37.6	38.0

From M. L. Pollock and A. S. Jackson with permission (personal communication)

TABLE 5. Relative body fat from the sum of six skinfolds in adult men 40 years of age and older

Sum of chest, thigh, suprailium, abdomen, triceps, and subscapula skinfolds

Sum of 6 Skinfolds	AGE TO THE LAST YEAR							
	41 to 43	44 to 46	47 to 49	50 to 52	53 to 55	56 to 58	59 to 61	62 and older
17– 23	4.1	4.5	4.9	5.3	5.7	6.1	6.5	6.9
24– 30	5.5	5.9	6.3	6.7	7.1	7.5	7.9	8.3
31– 37	6.9	7.3	7.7	8.1	8.5	8.9	9.3	9.7
38– 44	8.3	8.7	9.1	9.5	9.9	10.3	10.7	11.1
45– 51	9.6	10.0	10.4	10.8	11.2	11.6	12.0	12.4
52– 58	10.9	11.3	11.7	12.1	12.5	12.9	13.3	13.7
59– 65	12.2	12.6	13.0	13.4	13.8	14.2	14.6	15.0
66– 72	13.4	13.8	14.2	14.6	15.0	15.4	15.8	16.2
73– 79	14.7	15.1	15.5	15.9	16.3	16.7	17.1	17.5
80– 86	15.9	16.3	16.7	17.1	17.5	17.9	18.3	18.7
87– 93	17.0	17.4	17.8	18.2	18.6	19.0	19.4	19.8
94–100	18.2	18.6	19.0	19.4	19.8	20.2	20.6	21.0
101–107	19.3	19.7	20.1	20.5	20.9	21.3	21.7	22.1
108–114	20.3	20.7	21.1	21.5	21.9	22.3	22.7	23.1
115–121	21.4	21.8	22.2	22.6	23.0	23.4	23.8	24.2
122–128	22.4	22.8	23.2	23.6	24.0	24.4	24.8	25.2
129–135	23.4	23.8	24.2	24.6	25.0	25.4	25.8	26.2
136–142	24.4	24.8	25.2	25.6	26.0	26.4	26.8	27.2
143–149	25.3	25.7	26.1	26.5	26.9	27.3	27.7	28.1
150–156	26.2	26.6	27.0	27.4	27.8	28.2	28.6	29.0
157–163	27.1	27.5	27.9	28.3	28.7	29.1	29.5	29.9
164–170	28.0	28.4	28.8	29.2	29.6	30.0	30.4	30.8
171–177	28.8	29.2	29.6	30.0	30.4	30.8	31.2	31.6
178–184	29.6	30.0	30.4	30.8	31.2	31.6	32.0	32.4
185–191	30.3	30.7	31.1	31.5	31.9	32.3	32.7	33.1
192–198	31.1	31.5	31.9	32.3	32.7	33.1	33.5	33.9
199–205	31.8	32.2	32.6	33.0	33.4	33.8	34.2	34.6
206–212	32.5	32.9	33.3	33.7	34.1	34.5	34.9	35.3
213–219	33.1	33.5	33.9	34.3	34.7	35.1	35.5	35.9
220–226	33.8	34.2	34.6	35.0	35.4	35.8	36.2	36.6
227–233	34.4	34.8	35.2	35.6	36.0	36.4	36.8	37.2
234–240	34.9	35.3	35.7	36.1	36.5	36.9	37.3	37.7
241–247	35.5	35.9	36.3	36.7	37.1	37.5	37.9	38.3
248–254	36.0	36.4	36.8	37.2	37.6	38.0	38.4	38.8
255–261	36.5	36.9	37.3	37.7	38.1	38.5	38.9	39.3
262–268	36.9	37.3	37.7	38.1	38.5	38.9	39.3	39.7
269–275	37.3	37.7	38.1	38.5	38.9	39.3	39.7	40.1
276–282	37.7	38.1	38.5	38.9	39.3	39.7	40.1	40.5
283–289	38.1	38.5	38.9	39.3	39.7	40.1	40.5	40.9
290–296	38.4	38.8	39.2	39.6	40.0	40.4	40.8	41.2

From M. L. Pollock and A. S. Jackson with permission (personal communication)

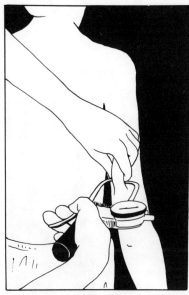

Triceps

FIGURE 6. Skinfold measurement at the triceps site

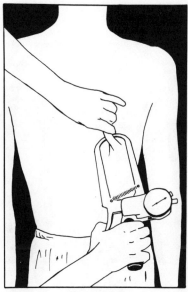

Scapula

FIGURE 7. Skinfold measurement at the scapula site

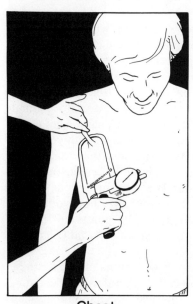

Chest

FIGURE 8. Skinfold measurement at the chest site

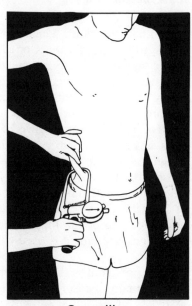

Suprailiac

FIGURE 9. Skinfold measurement at the suprailiac site

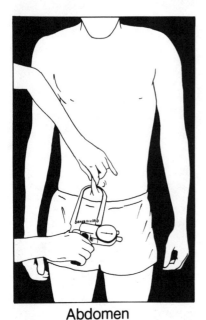

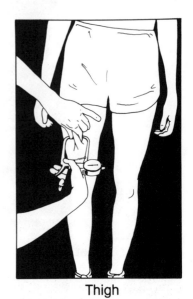

Abdomen

Thigh

FIGURE 10. Skinfold measurement at the abdominal site

FIGURE 11. Skinfold measurement at the thigh site

Another technique which can be used by anyone who doesn't have access to a skinfold caliper or to an underwater weighing facility employs only a tape measure. For men, the circumference of the waist, exactly at the level of the umbilicus, or belly button, is measured with the tape held firmly in the horizontal position, *i.e.,* do not allow the tape to slope upward or downward. The resulting measurement is used to estimate relative body fat from Figure 12 (page 35). Using a straight-edged device such as a ruler, line up your waist circumference or girth with your body weight, and your relative body fat is that point where the straight edge crosses the percent fat line. The illustration in Figure 12 demonstrates this calculation. With a body weight of 170 pounds and a waist circumference of 34 inches, the percent fat is estimated to be 18.0%. For women, the circumference of the hips is measured at its widest point and the subsequent measurement is used with height to estimate body fat (Figure 13, page 35).

How prevalent is the problem of obesity? Unfortunately, few studies have actually measured or estimated body fat; therefore, little data is available on the actual percentage of the American population that would meet the above definition of obesity. Depending on the various studies of overweight in the adult population, from 15% to 40% would be considered obese. Dr. Robert I. Levy, director of the National Heart, Lung, and

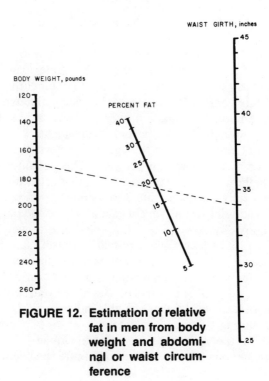

FIGURE 12. Estimation of relative fat in men from body weight and abdominal or waist circumference

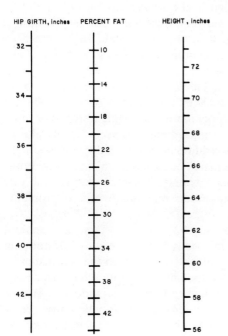

FIGURE 13. Estimation of relative fat in women from height and hip circumference

Blood Institute, has stated that obesity is a major health problem affecting at least 40,000,000, and perhaps as many as 90,000,000, adult Americans. He believes that obesity is the most common form of malnutrition in the United States today. Further, the American public spends over $10,000,000,000 a year in an attempt to combat the "battle of the bulge." The United States Public Health Service estimated in the year 1966, that of the American population over 30 years of age, from 25% to 46% are 20% or more above their best or ideal weight.

In both sexes, beyond the age of 25 years, the average individual will gain one pound of weight per year. This does not seem like much since your bathroom scales are usually not that accurate, and your body weight will typically fluctuate from 2 to 5 pounds during the course of a normal day. In addition to this weight gain of one pound per year, there is a loss of approximately one-quarter of a pound of lean weight each year resulting from a loss of lean tissue, primarily muscle and bone. Once the adult reduces his or her basic levels of exercise, there will be a decrease in lean tissue, similar to that seen when a broken arm or leg is placed in a cast. With a *net* gain of one pound of weight per year, but a loss of a quarter of a pound of lean weight per year, this indicates that the average American is accumulating 1¼ pounds of fat per year, or 37½ pounds of *extra* fat in 30 years, at the age of 55 years! No wonder the average middle-aged American comes home tired at night after a sedentary day's work at the office.

In a recent study (1978) published in the *American Journal of Public Health,* Professors Bruce Hannon and Timothy Lohman of the University of Illinois calculated the fossil fuel energy that would be required to supply the extra food calories just to maintain this excess body fat of our total American population. They estimated that there are 377,000,000 kilograms of excess fat in men and 667,000,000 kilograms of excess fat in women, yielding a total of 1,044,000,000 kilograms or 2,300,000,000 pounds of excess fat. The actual energy saved by dieting to reach optimal weight and the savings in energy resulting from lowered food intake to support the optimal body weight, would be more than sufficient to supply the annual residential electrical demands of Boston, Chicago, San Francisco, and Washington, D.C. When expressed in these terms, one can only begin to grasp the significance and magnitude of the problems associated with an obese society.

What is the basic cause of obesity? Over the years, the general population has been led to believe that obesity is the result of gluttony on the one hand, or glandular malfunction on the other. In the last instance, the responsibility is taken away from the individual and the obese condition is blamed on factors beyond the control of the individual. It is now recognized that obesity has many origins—including heredity, early over-nutrition, physical inactivity, social factors, psychological factors, and endocrine and rare syndromes. Of these factors, physical inactivity appears to be the most important for several reasons. First, with physical activity you have an additional expenditure of calories. Second, the regulation of appetite and food intake appears to be dependent on certain levels of physical activity. Without adequate activity, the body seems to lose the ability to fine tune the appetite, and extra, unneeded calories are consumed.

What are the ultimate consequences of obesity? The obese individual is at an increased risk for a number of serious medical problems. While hypertension is most closely associated with obesity, obesity has also been related to an increased risk for coronary artery disease, venous thrombosis, thrombophlebitis, diabetes, hyperlipidemia (elevated blood fats), hyperuricemia (possibly leading to gout), gastrointestinal disorders, respiratory disorders, kidney disease, and gallbladder disease. The obese individual is also at an increased risk for arthritis, surgery, accidents of all types, and, finally, the obese individual suffers from discrimination, emotional disorders, and restricted life-styles.

Anxiety and Depression

Anxiety and depression are two undesirable psychological states that have reached pandemic proportions in the United States in recent years. Emotional disturbance may be the cause of more marital, professional, and social distress than most organic diseases combined. Anxiety can be defined as a vague feeling of nervousness, apprehension, and uncertainty, and is similar to the feelings associated with fear. The feeling of anxiety, however, is frequently not associated with a specific cause or threat. It can produce confusion, and distorted perceptions of time and space, and distortion of motivation and meanings of events. It can hinder learning and normal mental processes through lowering of concentration, impairing memory, and decreasing the ability to relate one item to another. Depression is characterized by a sense of hopelessness, self-depreciation, bitterness, regret, and a slowing of emotional responses as well as mental and body functioning. It has been estimated that over 50% of all patients hospitalized with emotional illness have been diagnosed as suffering from various depression disorders.

The causes of anxiety and depression are numerous and often times vague. The physical fitness levels of individuals with emotional or mental disorders is typically low. Whether this is a possible cause or a consequence of the disorder has not been well established. Anxiety and depression are generally of a fairly mild nature with few consequences if treated early. Left untreated, however, the individual can develop serious psychological disorders which can result in complete incapacitation, or even death.

Musculoskeletal Disease or Disability

Problems related to lower back pain constitute one of the most frequent medical complaints faced by physicians. It is estimated that 20% to 40% of our adult population have had in the past, or presently have, acute or chronic back pain. In the mid-1940s, clinics to investigate possible causes of low back pain were instituted at Columbia Presbyterian Medical Center in New York City, and at the New York University Institute of Physical Medicine and Rehabilitation. Approximately 5,000 individuals were seen by their staffs which included specialists in orthopedic surgery, neurosurgery, neurology, and internal medicine, among others. In addition to the conventional medical examination, all of these patients were given tests to determine relative muscle strength and flexibility of key postural muscles. Of those patients who had chronic back problems, nearly 80% exhibited muscle weakness or poor flexibility, and had no specific disease, lesion, or other medical anomaly that could account for this back problem. Tension and lack of physical activity were major contributing factors in most of these cases. It was concluded that exercise has a protective value in the prevention of back pain, directly by keeping posture muscles flexible and strong, and indirectly by its natural tranquilizing effect, controlling nervous tension.

Arthritis, or "rheumatism," is a disease of the joints characterized by pain and stiffness, and is sometimes crippling. Approximately 12,000,000 to 15,000,000 Americans suffer from the disease. Essentially, there are two different types of arthritis: *rheumatoid arthritis,* and *osteoarthritis.* Rheumatoid arthritis is of unknown origin but can strike early in life and progress rapidly to deformed joints and general crippling. Osteoarthritis is far more common, and appears to be a part of the normal aging process. As one grows older, the joints, like other parts of the body, deteriorate from constant use, or from previous injury. By the age of 60 years, from 80% to 90% of the population have some deterioration of the weight-bearing joints. When the deterioration progresses to the point where movement of these joints becomes painful or difficult, this is then referred to as osteoarthritis. Anything that increases ordinary stress and strain on the joints may bring on osteoarthritis, including overweight, poor posture, and occupations requiring continual use of the joints under conditions of dampness and cold.

There is an associated problem which is related to osteoarthritis, and that is the fact that there is a general reduction in the mass of bone in the body as one reaches 50 to 60 years of age. This is the result of a loss in bone mineral, primarily calcium, as well as in the bone matrix, *i.e.,* the structural component of bone which supports the bone mineral. While this has been referred to as adult *osteoporosis,* this is not a totally correct designation. In true osteoporosis, there is a loss only in bone mineral, while the matrix remains intact. The consequences of this reduction in bone mass are several. First, the total body height will decrease up to an inch or more. Second, the bones become weaker, or more brittle, and are, therefore, much more susceptible to fracture. Once fractured, the bones heal very slowly, and because of the extended period of immobilization, particularly for weight-bearing bones, the individual frequently undergoes considerable deterioration of all body systems, with death being a frequent consequence. This extreme is seen most often in those over 65 years of age. The causes of the loss of bone mass are not well understood at the present time. Diet, hormonal change, as in menopause, and decreased physical activity are the three factors considered to be the most important potential causes, either singularly or in combination.

2

Promoting an
Active Life-Style —
Choice or Necessity?

THE ROLE OF PHYSICAL ACTIVITY IN COMBATING HYPOKINETIC DISEASE

In the previous chapter, the role of physical inactivity was discussed as it related to the most prevalent of the hypokinetic diseases, *i.e.,* coronary artery disease, hypertension, obesity, anxiety and depression, and musculoskeletal diseases and disability. While physical inactivity was strongly linked to each of these diseases, this does not imply that by increasing physical activity you can prevent the disease or undergo successful rehabilitation if the disease is present. The health-related benefits of an active and vigorous life-style are somewhat controversial, or, at best, poorly understood. In this chapter, an attempt will be made to describe the role of increased physical activity on each of the hypokinetic diseases defined and discussed previously. Only then can you make a decision as to whether promoting an active life-style is a choice or a necessity!

Coronary Artery Disease

Physical inactivity has been listed as a risk factor for coronary artery disease. There are still some researchers and clinicians, however, who seriously question the need for exercise in the prevention of this disease. What does the available research have to offer with respect to linking physical activity to the prevention of heart attacks?

Most of the original research on exercise and heart disease was of an epidemiological nature; observing in large populations the differences in the rate of heart attack and death from heart attack, comparing "sedentary" and "active" groups. The first large-scale study of this type was reported in 1953, in the British medical journal *Lancet,* by Professor J. N. Morris and his colleagues from London. They first compared bus drivers and bus conductors on the London transport system's double-deckered buses, where the drivers were considered sedentary and the conductors active as they climbed the stairs throughout the day collecting fares. They found that the physically more active conductors had 50% fewer heart attacks, and the mortality from coronary artery disease was less than half as frequent in the conductors. Next, the same investigators compared postal workers who delivered mail with less active postal service clerks and found essentially the same results, *i.e.,* the sedentary group was at a much higher risk.

It must be mentioned, before going any further with this line of evidence, that these types of studies do not necessarily demonstrate absolute cause-effect relationships. Taking the bus driver-bus conductor study as an illustration, upon further analysis of their data, Morris and his associates published an additional paper titled "Physique of Busmen: The Epidemiology of Uniforms." In this paper they found that for any given height, the bus drivers upon entry into the transport system were fitted with trousers that were at least one inch greater in waist circumference than the conductors. The drivers were also found to have higher serum cholesterol and blood pressure levels. Since the drivers were not the same as the conductors when they entered employment, it is difficult to determine if exercise played a significant role in reducing the number and severity of heart attacks, or whether this reduction was the result of their initial differences in two of the three primary risk factors, cholesterol and blood pressure, in addition to possible differences in total body fat.

Over the next 20 years, many additional studies of a similar nature were conducted, comparing the rate of heart attacks and deaths from heart attacks in active and sedentary populations. In over twenty studies during this period, only one failed to confirm that those who were sedentary in their occupation were at a higher risk than those who were active. Again, however, the problems associated with such an approach are many. What about those individuals who are totally sedentary in their occupations, yet may be quite active in their leisure time? They would traditionally be classified as sedentary, yet they may be getting far more exercise and activity than the individual in the active occupation who is relatively sedentary once he or she has left his job.

To overcome the above objections and to better control for other factors that can confuse the interpretation of the results of these population studies, Professor Morris and his associates studied the risk of heart attack in nearly 17,000 British male executive-grade civil servants, 40 to 64 years of age, in relation to leisure-time activity patterns. In this study, the subjects had similar on-the-job physical activity requirements, but they did differ markedly in their leisure-time activity levels. They found that in those who exercised vigorously in their leisure time, the relative risk of developing coronary disease was about a third of those men who were considered sedentary, or the risk was approximately three times greater for those in the sedentary group.

A fascinating study was reported in 1970, in which the Harvard School of Public Health and the Trinity College School of Medicine in Dublin, Ireland, collaborated to investigate 1,994 middle-aged men, including over 500 pairs of brothers, one of which lived in Ireland and the other in Boston. Since there is a substantially higher mortality rate from coronary artery disease in Massachusetts than in Ireland, an attempt was made to isolate which factors might be placing the American brothers in a higher risk category. They found that the intake of calories, complex carbohydrates, magnesium, and fluoride were higher in Ireland, while the proportion of calories derived from fat and saturated fat, serum cholesterol levels, blood pressures, and smoking habits did not differ markedly. They concluded that increased physical activity appears to be important in reducing the risk of coronary artery disease in Ireland.

Additional studies have been reported by Paffenbarger and his associates on their longitudinal research with longshoremen in the San Francisco Bay area, and on graduates of Harvard University. These studies strongly support the recurring finding that the sedentary individual is at a substantially greater risk for the early development of coronary artery disease when compared to the active individual.

Again, since cause-effect cannot be absolutely demonstrated with studies of this nature, it is also necessary to look at alternative ways of demonstrating a link between physical activity and the prevention of coronary artery disease. One approach is to determine the influence of physical activity on the other risk factors for coronary artery disease. In a comprehensive study of approximately 3,000 men, with an average age of 44.6 years, Cooper and his associates at the Institute of Aerobics Research in Dallas, Texas, reported that those men who had the highest levels of physical fitness had lower resting heart rates, body weights, percent body fats, blood serum levels of cholesterol and triglycerides, glucose, and systolic blood pressures. Thus, the more fit the individual, the lower his risk for coronary artery disease.

While the above study was of a cross-sectional nature—i.e., the subjects were observed only once—longitudinal studies, where individuals are actually placed on exercise programs, and studied before and after, tend to confirm these results. Exercise programs have been shown to reduce blood pressure in those individuals who are classified as hypertensive, to reduce blood serum levels of cholesterol (minimal change) and triglycerides, to reduce stress and anxiety, to reduce relative and absolute body fat, and to help in the management of the diabetic patient. Also, the

American Cancer Society and other groups or agencies have used exercise in their programs for smoking control, and have found exercise to be a good substitute therapy.

Even though the cross-sectional and longitudinal studies provide additional insight into the exercise-heart attack relationship, they still do not provide absolute, irrefutable proof that physical activity is important in preventing heart attacks, and in increasing the chances of survival from heart attacks. While considerable evidence is accumulating each day in support of vigorous exercise, it continues to be of an indirect, rather than direct, nature. Samuel M. Fox, III, M.D., prominent cardiologist, in the *American Journal of Cardiology* recognizes the present dilemma and has proposed the following solution. Rather than either accepting or rejecting a theory on the basis of absolute proof or not, he feels that it is acceptable to discuss additional levels of acceptance of preventive or therapeutic approaches: (1) proved beyond reasonable doubt; (2) of probable benefit, but not above question; (3) a prudent action—on the basis of a good chance of benefit, and an acceptably low hazard; and (4) promising, but more good data is needed. At the time this article was written (1969), Dr. Fox concluded that it is prudent to include increased habitual physical activity in a program to prevent or manage non-acute coronary heart disease. Some 10 years later, it would seem appropriate to move up one more rung on the ladder and conclude that exercise is of probable benefit, but not above question.

The major reason for taking a more positive stand for exercise has come from a series of studies conducted over the past few years. One always feels more comfortable in supporting a particular theory if the basic mechanisms can be identified through which the theory can operate. Prior to the last few years, there was little evidence to support a mechanism by which vigorous physical activity could alter one's risk for heart attack. Now, these recent studies are starting to uncover that possible mechanism. Cholesterol, implicated as a primary risk factor, is a fatty substance which is manufactured in the liver and consumed in the diet, and which builds up on the inner wall of the arteries, causing a narrowing of the channel through which the blood must flow. Since cholesterol is not soluble in blood—*i.e.*, it will always separate out and rise to the top—if it is to be transported in the blood it must be packaged in a form acceptable in the blood. Cholesterol is carried through the blood by a series of molecules called *lipoproteins*. There are four major lipoproteins. The *chylomicrons* are the largest and the lightest lipoproteins, consisting of approximately 80% to 95% triglyceride, 2% to 7% cholesterol, and the remainder is phospholipid and protein. *Very low density lipoproteins* (VLDL) are the next largest and lightest lipoproteins, and are composed of approximately 15% cholesterol, 60% triglyceride, with the remainder phospholipid and protein. *Low density lipoproteins* (LDL) are a smaller but more dense lipoprotein which are composed of nearly 50% cholesterol, 5% to 10% triglyceride, and a balance of phospholipid and protein. Finally, the *high density lipoprotein* (HDL) is the smallest of the lipoproteins and contains approximately 20% cholesterol, 5% triglyceride, and a balance of phospholipid and protein.

Of what significance is the above to coronary artery disease, and specifically to the role of exercise in this disease? Recent studies have found that those individuals with very low levels of HDL and high levels of LDL are at an extremely high risk for heart attack. Conversely, high HDL levels appear to provide a degree of protection from heart disease. In fact, HDL levels may be the single most important risk factor for predicting coronary artery disease. Thus, one can have normal, or even relatively high, total cholesterol levels, but if it is in the form of HDL cholesterol, it will be a positive, not a negative risk factor!

To date, there have been only three ways identified to alter HDL cholesterol levels, hormones (birth control pills), moderate intake of alcohol, and vigorous, endurance exercise. It appears that exercise may exert the greatest influence on elevating HDL cholesterol levels, thus providing possible protection from heart attack! How does HDL cholesterol provide protection? It is presently thought that HDL affixes itself to the arterial wall and actually removes cholesterol from the arterial wall and transports this cholesterol back to the liver where it is either stored or excreted. Thus, HDL appears to be a cholesterol scavenger, removing rather than depositing cholesterol in the inside lining of the arterial wall. Dr. Peter Wood and his associates at Stanford University have pioneered much of this early work relating endurance activity to elevations in HDL cholesterol levels, and to reductions in LDL cholesterol. While there are still many unanswered questions, there is now a strong case that can be made for promoting vigorous exercise of an endurance nature in the prevention of heart attacks.

One word of caution, less we get too carried away. Direct, absolute proof of the exercise-heart attack prevention link is still missing. We should be wary of enthusiasts who make claims that if one is able to run distances such as a marathon, that virtual immunity from fatal heart attacks is assured. Thomas J. Bassler, M.D., a pathologist and an active marathoner, has stated, "As no cases of fatal atherosclerosis have been documented in marathon finishers of any age, it follows that such activity confers virtual immunity from fatal heart attacks," and that "immunity to a heart attack coexists with the ability to cover 42 kilometers on foot." Unfortunately, Dr. Bassler's statements are totally conjecture at this time, and are not based on scientific fact. While the motives of individuals who make such claims are probably pure and are an attempt to promote an active life-style in a sedentary population, such claims only serve to confuse the basic issues, and, in some cases, actually work to discourage the sedentary individual from exercising, since he has difficulty even visualizing the walking of a mile. Jogging or running 26.2 miles would seem to be totally impossible.

Before leaving this discussion on coronary artery disease, it is encouraging to note that there has actually been a steady decrease in the mortality rate (deaths/100,000 population) for coronary heart disease since 1968, a decrease of over 30% in the past 30 years, 60% of which has occurred between 1968 and 1978 (Figure 14, below). The absolute number of cardiovascular deaths also fell below 1,000,000 in 1975 and 1976 for the first time since 1963. It is unclear at this time what changes have taken place that have led to this dramatic reversal. Dr. Robert I.

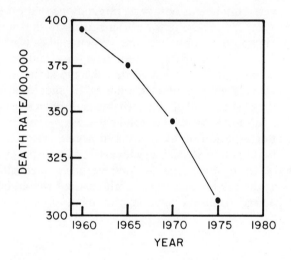

FIGURE 14. Decline in death rate from cardiovascular disease since the year 1960

Levy, director of the National Institutes of Health's National Heart, Lung, and Blood Institute, has listed the following as major clinical advances in the treatment of cardiovascular disease in a recent article in *Modern Concepts of Cardiovascular Disease:*

• Advanced diagnostic, screening, and monitoring techniques
• Artificial replacement and repair of diseased blood vessels
• Surgical repair of the heart
• Concepts of intensive care
• Drug therapies for hypertension
• Chemotherapies and antibiotics for treatment of heart disease
• Assessment of risk factors

It is likely that this increased public awareness of and attention to the risk factors has made a major contribution, with a renewed interest in exercise playing a role which has still yet to be defined, but one which many feel is very important.

Hypertension

The role of exercise in treating hypertension is somewhat better understood. Many of the early studies observing the influence of regular endurance exercise on resting blood pressure found little or no change in either systolic or diastolic blood pressure following weeks to months of vigorous exercise. It was only later that it became apparent that most of these studies were conducted, observing populations that essentially had normal blood pressure. Thus, it wasn't surprising to find normal blood pressures staying approximately the same. When studies were conducted on individuals who were truly hypertensive—*i.e.,* elevated systolic and/or diastolic pressure—they found that the blood pressure returned toward normal levels with endurance training. It should be mentioned, however, that the best control of hypertension is through a combination of diet, restricting salt intake as well as total calories, weight reduction, and exercise. If, after a period of six months to a year, the blood pressure levels have not dropped to satisfactory levels, it may be necessary for the patient's physician to prescribe anti-hypertensive medication. In all cases, however, the total management of the patient should be under the direct supervision of his or her personal physician.

Obesity

It is commonly thought that exercise is a very inefficient method of weight loss and weight control. Two basic arguments have surfaced over the years to support this concept. The first argument states that it takes far too much exercise to lose a single pound of fat. Numerous examples have been given to illustrate this point, such as you must chop wood for 7 hours, walk 35 miles, or climb a 10-foot staircase 1,000 times. The purpose of these examples is to show the foolishness of trying to lose weight through exercise. The second argument states that exercise only serves to increase the appetite, and this increase in calories consumed will be equal to or even exceed the number of calories used to perform the exercise.

Both of these arguments are misleading and erroneous. In fact, research has proven that exercise may be the most efficient way to lose weight and also results in weight losses of a more permanent nature. As we stated earlier, inactivity is a major cause of obesity in the United States. Thus, exercise must also be recognized as a significant factor in any program of weight reduction or control. The following factors must be considered when evaluating the efficacy of an exercise program in promoting losses in body fat.

First, it requires the use of approximately 3,500 calories to lose a pound of fat. This caloric value of a pound of fat will differ considerably from one individual to the next, and even within an individual depending on the composition of the weight loss as well as a number of factors which will not be discussed. For purposes of illustration, 3,500 calories per pound of fat is acceptable. This 3,500 calorie deficit can be accomplished in one of three ways: dieting, exercise, or a combination of diet and exercise. By taking one buttered slice of bread out of the diet each day (approximately 100 calories), the individual would lose one pound of fat in 35 days, providing everything else remained constant. Likewise, one pound of fat could be lost in 35 days by walking or jogging one mile each day (approximately 100 calories expended per mile), again assuming all other factors remained constant. By combining this modest decrease in food intake and increase in activity level, it would be possible to lose the same pound of fat in only half of that time, *i.e.*, 17½ days. One could speed up the process of fat loss considerably. As an example, by walking 5 miles a day (500 calories) and decreasing food intake by 500 calories per day, it would be possible to have a total caloric deficit of 1,000 calories per day, which would allow the loss of one pound of fat every 3½ days, or two pounds of fat loss per week!

However, the above approach doesn't appeal to the general American population, for we are a society that is geared for the immediate—the "now generation." We are accustomed to having whatever we want, whenever we want it. The concept of waiting while one earns and saves to purchase something of considerable value to that individual has become old and outdated. One just simply borrows money—*e.g.*, "instant cash"—and he or she can have whatever it is that is desired almost immediately. This same philosophy applies to almost all walks of life. The young woman who is 30 pounds above desirable weight, and who is invited to the big dance of the year which is just one month away, decides it is time to lose that weight so she will have a desirable appearance on the night of the dance. The weight loss goal of 30 pounds is admirable, but the time sequence is totally unreasonable, *i.e.*, one pound weight loss per day. The "paunchy" middle-aged male who is due to return for a reunion of his high school graduating class is confronted with the problem of being 50 pounds overweight, and with the reunion only six weeks away, he decides that it is time to get back into shape. Again, this goal is noble but the expectations unrealistic.

The American population spends billions of dollars each year in combating the "battle of the bulge," only in most instances to face a losing battle. Weight which is rapidly lost is frequently regained even more rapidly. Dr. Jean Mayer, president of Tufts University, and world-famous nutritionist, formerly of Harvard University, has used the term to describe this phenomenom as the "rhythm method" of girth control. Such repetitive patterns of weight loss and weight gain are psychologically destructive to the individual and can also have serious medical implications over time.

What is the basic cause of the failures noted above, and how does this relate to the topic under discussion, exercise in weight reduction and weight control? The major cause of failure in most weight loss programs relates to the urgency factor; once the decision is made to lose the weight, the desired weight loss must be accomplished immediately. This frequently leads to a search for the latest fad diet. Unfortunately, nutrition is an area which has spawned many self-proclaimed experts, so if one has the appropriate credentials, such as an M.D. or Ph.D. degree, this allows that individual license to develop the next wonder diet in which it is claimed to be possible to lose 5 to 10 pounds per week with only "minor" modifications in one's life-style. In the past, we have heard that "calories don't count," and that you can eat as much as you want, providing you eat only certain foods. Most of us even know of friends or relatives who have lost 5 to 10 pounds per week using one of the modern miracle diets. Yet, the results remain basically the same, quick weight loss and rapid weight gain once the dieting period has ended.

The public has been misled into believing that quick weight loss schemes really work, when in fact they typically don't. The reasons are very simple. Using 3,500 calories as the equivalent of one pound of weight loss, it would be possible to lose no more than one pound of weight per day if one were to totally abstain from food intake, and expend 3,500 calories every 24 hours. The average adult male and female who engage in moderate levels of activity need approximately 2,800 and 2,000 calories, respectively, to maintain their body weight; *i.e.*, such a diet over an extended period of time will result in neither a weight loss or a weight gain. This figure was established in 1968 by the Food and Nutrition Board of the National Academy of Science's National Research Council. Thus, to attain a one pound per day loss of weight, the average male would have to use 700 additional calories in exercise (equivalent to walking or jogging 7 miles) as well as to refrain from eating. The average female would have to expend an extra 1,500 calories in exercise (walking or jogging 15 miles) in addition to abstaining from food. It is obvious that these are totally unrealistic approaches to weight loss, yet how can we explain the 5 to 10 pound weight losses some individuals experience in a one-week period of time?

Most rapid-weight-loss diets have one thing in common—they allow only a modest intake of carbohydrates. Carbohydrates constitute approximately 60% of the normal mixed diet. When carbohydrate intake is lowered to levels of 10% or less of the total food intake, combined with a reduction in total food intake, the body starts to utilize its own carbohydrate stores in the liver and muscles. When you store a gram of carbohydrate in the liver or muscles, you store along with it approximately 3 grams of water. When you use a gram of carbohydrate from the body stores, you will lose 3 grams of water. Thus, as the body stores of carbohydrate are being reduced as a result of a low-calorie diet deficient in carbohydrate, there will be a substantial loss of body water. Also, additional water is lost as a result of the greater utilization of fat, which results in an increased production of *ketone bodies,* which are by-products of fat metabolism. *Ketosis,* or an elevation of ketone bodies in the blood, frequently results and is characterized by a distinct acetone odor on the breath. The ketone bodies will spill into the urine; thus, many of these diets encourage self-administered, periodic testing of the urine with ketone sticks to keep this condition under control. Prolonged periods of ketosis can have substantial detrimental effects on the body. The combined effects of ketosis and utilization of the body's carbohydrate stores results in a substantial loss of water. Thus, the large losses of weight that occur within the first few weeks of dieting are essentially losses of body fluids, not body fat! In fact, several studies have demonstrated that from 60% to 70% of this weight loss is from the lean body tissue, which includes the body fluids.

For the average female, it is literally impossible to lose more than 3 pounds of fat per week, even under the most extreme conditions. If the average female who normally consumes 2,000 calories to maintain body weight were to fast for a period of one week, which is not a recommended procedure, she would theoretically lose the fat equivalent of 2,000 calories per day, or nearly 0.6 of a pound per day (2,000 cal. ÷ 3,500 cal./lb. = 0.57 lb.). However, when you reduce your food intake to starvation or near-starvation levels, the body reduces its energy needs by 25% to 30%. Thus, where the body was requiring 2,000 calories per day with normal food intake, it requires substantially less when it is under the stress of inadequate food intake, *i.e.,* 1,400 to 1,500 calories. The equivalent amount of fat lost per day is reduced accordingly to approximately 0.4 of a pound, or 2.8 pounds per week with total starvation!

Referring back to the previous discussion, it was shown that by combining diet and exercise, it was possible to achieve a deficit of 1,000 calories per day, which is equivalent to approximately 2 pounds of fat loss per week. While this may appear to be the slow approach to weight loss, it is the most sensible approach. Losses of lean tissue are minimal, and research evidence indicates that the losses are more likely to be of a permanent nature, *i.e.,* not likely to be regained over time. This last point is an extremely critical one, as the success or failure of any weight loss program should be measured only after a period of several years have passed from the time that the desired weight was attained. If the weight loss has been maintained, then the program can be considered a success. The reason the rapid-weight-loss programs so often result in failure is the fact that once a desired weight is achieved, the individual typically will return to a normal diet, which is typically high in carbohydrates. The water which was lost during the dieting period is quickly regained, often in a matter of only a few days. Thus, the individual's weight literally jumps back to its previous level, and the diet is considered a failure.

Exercise is, therefore, an essential part of any sound weight reduction and weight control program. While it does take considerable activity to achieve a significant weight loss, chances are it will be a permanent weight loss. Many research studies have confirmed the fact that it is possible to lose approximately a quarter of a pound of fat per week from an exercise program that requires no more than 3 days per week, 30 minutes per day. This would be approximately the equivalent of walking or jogging 9 miles per week. While this doesn't seem like much, this rate of fat loss would result in a total loss in one year of 13 pounds, and this is from exercise alone. These results can be even more substantial when *moderate* dieting is included. Doesn't exercise increase the appetite so you take in more food? Several studies on humans as well as animals have shown that moderate levels of activity even tend to decrease one's appetite. Individuals who have started exercise programs, such as jogging, find that if they exercise just prior to their biggest meal, which is typically dinner, they will not eat as much—the appetite is just not there. Increasing evidence is accumulating which is suggesting that the body must have a certain basic level of exercise before it is able to regulate appetite, and thus food intake, to match the energy expenditure. If activity levels drop below this basic level, the body loses its ability to "fine-tune" the appetite, with a resulting increase in food consumption above that which is needed. This inability to fine-tune may result in only a seemingly small imbalance of 10 calories per day (approximately one potato chip), but over a period of one year this adds an excess of 3,600 calories per year, or the equivalent of an added pound of fat.

When using an exercise program to complement dieting in weight reduction, it is important to remember that as we get older we lose lean tissue, primarily muscle and bone mass, as we discussed earlier. This is the result of an increasingly sedentary life-style. However, when one starts to exercise, this process reverses itself and the body tends to gain lean weight. Thus, it is not uncommon to find little or no change in the scale or total body weight over the first few weeks to months that the individual is on the program. This is a normal phenomenon and should be expected. Fat weight is being lost, but lean weight is being gained in approximately the same amount. This will leave one with the impression that the program is a failure, since there is little or no change in scale weight, yet fat is being lost. The individual should not use the scale as his or her means of judging progress over the first few months. A far better indicator of those changes that are taking place is the way one's clothes fit, for there is a redistribution of the weight, leading to a much more desirable figure or physique. The increase in lean body weight will tend to level off after the first few months in the program. At this point, there will be a detectable reduction in body weight as fat weight will continue to decrease.

Lastly, in addition to a formal exercise program, attempting to be more active in all aspects of one's life can also result in substantial dividends. One study noted that when switching from manual to electric typewriters, secretaries tended to put on small amounts of additional weight. While a return to the manual typewriter is not advocated, this study does show that even small increases or decreases in activity level can have a significant influence on our body fat levels. Most individuals spend at least eight hours per day at work, or approximately 50% or their waking hours, or a third to a fourth of their life. Thus, any extra activity that can be structured into the work day on a regular basis will have an influence over an extended period of time. Taking stairs instead of elevators or escalators, parking two or three blocks farther from work than where you normally park, or just performing your daily activities in a more active manner will all work toward the common goal of increasing caloric expenditure and decreasing elevated fat stores to more normal levels. Our American society must begin to think of the treatment of obesity as a long-term project, and anyone who wishes to lose even small amounts of weight should project a weight loss goal of no more than one or two pounds per week, and even this should be done with the approval of the individual's family physician.

Anxiety and Depression

A low physical fitness profile is frequently found in patients with various mental diseases or illnesses. Is there a direct cause-effect relationship, or do these two facts simply coexist, both the result of another factor which has not been identified? If there is a direct cause-effect relationship, which factor is the causative factor? Often, inactivity is the result of the disease itself, as in schizophrenics and other psychotic patients who are characterized by a significant general passivity, impaired mobility, lack of communication, and a tendency to autistic thinking and regression which results in an even greater reduction in physical endurance capacity and muscular strength. Also, in various neurotic states, there is a tendency to avoid physical activity for fear that that activity will precipitate serious medical consequences, *e.g.,* fast heart rate leading to a fatal heart attack. In addition, certain drugs used in the treatment of mental disorders (psychotropic drugs) have side effects which would tend to reduce normal levels of physical activity. There is little, if any, direct evidence that indicates that reduced levels of physical activity leading to low levels of physical fitness are related to the onset of the various mental diseases. It is quite possible that physical inactivity, per se, is not the specific cause, but creates an environment which increases the likelihood of that individual developing that particular mental disorder. Additional research will be necessary to determine if exercise or the lack of exercise plays a specific role in either preventing (exercise) or causing (lack of exercise) specific mental diseases. In the meantime, a growing body of knowledge is pointing to the importance of cardiovascular endurance exercises in the treatment of mental disorders.

In several early research investigations, investigators reported reductions in tension and anxiety with increased levels of physical activity. Unfortunately, these early studies were not sufficiently controlled to the point where a direct cause-effect relationship could be assumed. Professor Herbert A. deVries and his colleagues at the University of Southern California found through a series of studies that vigorous physical activity produced a significant reduction in muscular tension as evaluated by electrodes which monitored the electrical activity of the underlying muscles. Furthermore, they found that exercise was even more effective in reducing muscular tension than a commonly employed tranquilizer. Professor William P. Morgan, from the University of Wisconsin, in summarizing the research in the area of exercise and its role in reducing anxiety and tension, makes the important observation that similar reductions have been noted with the use of such techniques as progressive relaxation, biofeedback, meditation, and hypnosis.

Other studies have demonstrated that exercise must be of a relatively vigorous nature, approaching 70% to 80% of the individual's capacity, in order to achieve reductions in anxiety. Where exercise was of a relatively low intensity, or of short duration, anxiety levels were not altered. There does appear to be a threshold level which one must achieve in order to maximize the benefits of the exercise relative to anxiety reduction.

With respect to depression, several studies have recently been published which indicate that endurance conditioning results in a reduction in levels of depression. Dr. John H. Greist, and his associates at the University of Wisconsin, conducted a study of running as a treatment for moderate depression. Males and females, 18 to 30 years of age who were clinically diagnosed as having moderate depression, were randomly assigned to either ten sessions of time-limited psychotherapy, focusing on immediate changes people can make to help themselves feel better; or to time-unlimited psychotherapy, which is an insight-oriented, dynamic psychotherapy; or running treatment. They found that six of the eight patients on the running program were essentially well within the first three weeks and remained that way for the duration of the treatment period and the subsequent follow-up period. For the running group as a whole, the results compared favorably with those of patients undergoing psychotherapy.

Dr. Robert S. Brown, a practicing psychiatrist at the University of Virginia, Charlottesville, and his associates found similar results in a much larger population. They found substantial reductions in depression scores in those who jogged for a period of ten weeks, but little or no change in those who played softball or tennis. Similar to those studies reviewed earlier with exercise and anxiety, this suggests a certain threshold of activity that must be achieved before alterations can be obtained. In a second phase of this same study, Dr. Brown and his associates selected 101 university students who were clinically depressed and placed 91 of them into an exercise program of running, with the remaining 10 serving as non-exercising controls. An additional 406 students with no symptoms of depression were placed into the running program, and 54 students with no symptoms of depression served as non-exercising controls. Following the ten-week exercise program there was a substantial reduction in depression scores in both the normal and the depressed groups who jogged, while no changes were noted for either the normal or depressed groups who refrained from exercise. In addition, the negative affective states of anger/hostility, fatigue/inertia, and tense/anxious were subsequently reduced and the positive affective states of cheerfulness, energy, and activation were significantly increased in the depressed subjects who jogged.

It is a common finding that individuals who are involved in a program of regular physical activity of an endurance nature have an increased sense of well-being. There is definitely a sense of "feeling better" that accompanies such an activity program. In fact, Dr. William Glasser, in his book *Positive Addiction,* has reported that joggers or runners who exercise 30 to 60 minutes per day, 4 days a week or more, frequently become addicted to this routine. If illness, injury, travel, or some other interruption disrupts their exercise routine, these individuals actually go through withdrawal-like symptoms! For the non-exerciser, it is difficult to comprehend how vigorous exercise could provide such pleasure.

From the above, it does appear that vigorous physical activity of an endurance nature does promote good mental health, particularly in the areas of anxiety and depression. While many of those studies which have been conducted to date could be criticized for being poorly controlled or improperly designed, the evidence is sufficient to allow one to conclude that a healthy mind is typically found in a healthy body, and that physical activity of an endurance nature will improve the health of the mind as well as the body.

Musculoskeletal Disease and Disability

While problems of the lower back are a major medical complaint of a substantial percentage of our adult population, most of these problems, approximately 80%, can be linked to a combination of reduced range of movement in the various joints of the body (inflexibility) and inadequate muscular strength to properly support the structure and weight of the body. Fortunately, these are problems which can be corrected with the appropriate selection of flexibility and strength exercises. In one study, where 233 patients with lower back complaints were followed for a period of approximately 8 years, 82% reported substantial therapeutic improvement following an exercise program which emphasized the development of strength and flexibility. Even patients with osteoarthritic changes greatly increased their functional potential with adequate exercise. The National Y.M.C.A. has recently instituted a program in over 700 Y.M.C.A.'s around the country for treating back pain due to muscle deficiency which is referred to as "The Y's Way to a Healthy Back." This program emphasizes stretching and strength-type exercise, and has produced excellent improvement in 29%, good improvement in 36%, and fair improvement in 25% of a sample of 421 participants representing 19 Y.M.C.A.'s.

With respect to lower back problems, this appears to be one area where improvement can occur within a relatively short period of time, providing the condition is the result of inflexibility and weak musculature. Simple stretching and strengthening exercises done for 10 to 20 minutes per day can bring almost immediate relief, but the program must be maintained indefinitely or the problem will typically recur.

With respect to those changes in bone which result from aging—*e.g.,* osteoarthritis and osteoporosis—chronic exercise has been shown to provide limited if not substantial alterations in bone metabolism which appear to slow down the general progressive deterioration that results with aging. In a recent study of a group of older women, who averaged 82 years of age at the beginning of the study, 12 women exercised 3 days per week for 30 minutes per day performing light to moderate activity, and 17 women remained sedentary. At the end of 36 months, the control group of non-exercisers experienced a 2.5% decrease in bone mineral, while the exercise group actually experienced a 4.2% increase. It is known from a number of studies conducted on farm animals and humans that enforced periods of inactivity can lead to substantial decreases in bone mineral. This was a major concern when NASA was initially considering extended periods of space flight. Results from the early space flights indicated the astronauts were experiencing rather substantial losses in bone mineral following these periods of weightlessness in a confined environment. The extended missions, including SkyLab, made provisions for exercise on board the space vehicle or laboratory, to minimize changes in bone minerals as well as to reduce the possibility of general cardiovascular deconditioning. Bone apparently needs the stress of bearing the body weight in order to be maintained at optimal efficiency.

PREVENTIVE MEDICINE—A TOTAL APPROACH TO HEALTH CARE

From the preceding, it would appear prudent, if not essential, that exercise become an important addition to the life-style of the typically sedentary American, whether a young child or a senior citizen. For those who have established good exercise habits and enjoy what they are doing, they should be encouraged to continue, for exercise is a lifetime pursuit. One cannot engage in an exercise program for a period of weeks, months, or even years, and then stop to assume a sedentary life-style, expecting to live on the residual benefits of the previous activity. Many alterations in bodily function occur with physical activity which are beneficial to the total health of the individual. However, these benefits are quickly lost when activity is discontinued or interrupted for an extended period of time. For those individuals who have been sedentary, activity should be gradually included as a part of their daily schedule or routine. While it may seem impossible to crowd even more into an already over-committed schedule, and many may feel that they cannot justify this additional commitment as an efficient use of their time, the ultimate benefits to be derived from a regular program of vigorous activity may indeed make the exercise period the cornerstone of each day's activities. Factors such as improved self-image, with the accompanying improvement in self-confidence, the need for less sleep, the release of anxiety and tension, in addition to the general sense of well-being that accompanies a regular program of vigorous activity, will actually provide dividends in time that will far outweigh the minimal time investment required on a daily basis. In short, physical activity increases the overall efficiency of the body to a level where optimal function is achieved in nearly all aspects of life.

However, exercise is only one aspect of a total approach to health care. There are many other factors which, when combined, provide for optimal health, and contribute to *preventive medicine*. Over the past few years, the concept of preventive medicine has undergone a rather radical and important change. In the past, preventive medicine was essentially limited in concept to such essential practices as providing inoculations to prevent specific diseases, and the treatment of water and sewage to prevent the spread of various diseases. Recently, it has become increasingly apparent that the responsibility for health care can also be shared by the individual, *i.e.*, there is much every person can do to promote health and reduce the risk of disease and disability in their own lives. In addition to increasing physical activity, individuals can alter their diets, decrease or stop smoking, reduce alcohol intake to more reasonable levels, allow sufficient time for sleep, and reduce those factors in their present life-style which contribute to increased levels of emotional stress and anxiety.

Often, the individual recognizes a need for a drastic change in his or her life-style, either as a result of an existing health problem, or the feeling and fear of impending sickness. This is frequently the major motivator which results in these individuals undertaking an exercise program. While this in itself is not bad, all too often these same individuals have additional undesirable habits which should be altered, but they feel that exercise alone will provide them with an instant cure, allowing them to continue their other bad habits. This is not an uncommon pattern for those who have had heart attacks and are heavy smokers. These individuals will frequently join a cardiac rehabilitation program where they can start the process of physical reconditioning with the hope and expectation that this alone will resolve their heart problem, allowing them to continue smoking. To concentrate on only one risk factor to the exclusion of others which may be present is unwise. The total life-style of the individual must be evaluated, and attention should be given to all factors which place that individual at risk for any preventable disease.

An additional factor of importance to the total concept of preventive medicine is the periodic medical examination. It has been estimated that the risk of death from various preventable diseases can be reduced by 50% or more simply by having an annual or semi-annual medical examination. Properly conducted, the medical examination can identify various diseases in their early stages, providing a much better chance for total cure or control of the disease. Early detection procedures have been identified for coronary heart disease, hypertension, various forms of cancer, diabetes, and various respiratory diseases, among others. Too often, a disease is detected only in its terminal stages, and this reduces considerably the chances for survival. While no one wants to be told he or she has a serious disease or medical problem, it is far better to have advanced warning where corrective procedures can be instituted early in the course of the disease, thereby increasing the chances of survival and/or recovery to full health and a productive life.

At what age should one start having periodic medical examinations, and how frequently should these be administered? Undoubtedly, the best time to start with a comprehensive medical examination is early in life when health is at its peak. A comprehensive medical examination at age 20 to 25 years provides an excellent base-line examination which can serve as a reference for examinations later in life when the individual's health is starting to fail. There is considerable individual variation of normal values for just about all parameters measured in a medical examination. When an individual develops a specific disease or medical problem and his medical profile is measured against the population norms, it may be difficult, if not impossible, to establish an accurate diagnosis since the individual's values for any one test may fall within the rather broad range of values considered normal for that test, while being well out of line for what is normal for that individual. The base-line examination, taken at an early age during a period of optimal health, will provide an invaluable reference throughout life, enabling the comparison of all subsequent examinations to determine when any one test starts to vary from normal, as defined by that individual's normal range of variation for that specific test. A comprehensive medical examination every two or three years is recommended for those who have no specific complaints, up to the age of 35 to 45 years of age, at which point an annual examination is recommended. Preventive maintenance has been proven to minimize mechanical failures and to prolong the life of an automobile. A similar program of preventive maintenance is essential for promoting man's health and reducing the risk of serious disease and disability.

SECTION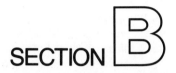

The Prescription
of Exercise for
Fitness and Sport

During the past decade a number of advances have been made in the exercise and sport sciences which have had a major influence on the development of safe and sound guidelines for the prescription of exercise. It wasn't too many years ago that exercise programs were initiated for the masses, with everyone performing the same activity and doing essentially the same sequence and intensity of performance. Individuals would line up by the rows to perform in unison an entire series of calisthenic-type exercises, followed by several laps around the gymnasium, an enthusiastic game of volleyball or basketball, several more laps around the gym, and then on to the showers. This was very typical of many of the Y.M.C.A., Y.W.C.A., or Jewish Community Center programs of the 1950s. At that time, these were considered excellent programs for the development of physical fitness and the promotion of health. Today, the prescription of exercise has developed into a science. Where all participants were provided with identical exercise programs in the past, it is now recognized that exercise must be prescribed on an individualized basis. It is also known that different sports and activities provide widely different benefits. In addition, the benefits of exercise have been proven to vary considerably with the intensity at which the individual plays an activity, in addition to the number of minutes per day and the number of days of the week the individual is involved.

This section presents a detailed examination of those factors which should be considered when initiating an exercise program. A thorough medical evaluation should precede any formal prescription of exercise.

59

The contents of such an evaluation will be described in addition to outlining those medical problems which would preclude formal exercise under any conditions, or where the risk is sufficiently great to indicate the need for a structured program under the close supervision of a physician. The essential ingredients of a sound, comprehensive exercise prescription are then outlined, followed by a discussion of appropriate warm-up, cool-down, and flexibility exercises; activities to promote cardiorespiratory fitness; training for strength, power, and muscular endurance; and finally the role of sport and recreational activities in the promotion of fitness and sport.

3

The Medical Evaluation
and Clearance
for Exercise

INTRODUCTION

It is relatively uncommon for the average individual to consult his private physician prior to starting an exercise program. However, it is now well documented that a certain percentage of individuals who assume they are healthy, with no apparent disease or risk for disease, will have on closer examination a serious medical problem that will: 1) dictate additional diagnostic procedures and further medical follow-up; 2) place limitations on the exercise prescription, including the possibility of allowing exercise only under the close supervision of a physician or a trained paramedical associate; or 3) preclude the prescription of exercise altogether. The percentage of those who would be identified as having a serious medical problem will vary considerably according to age. Probably fewer than 2% to 5% of those between the ages of 5 and 25 years would fall into this category. However, the older one is, the longer he has been sedentary, and the more undesirable health habits he has acquired over the years, the greater the risk of falling into this category of having a serious medical problem, or being at a higher risk for a serious medical problem. In a series of studies conducted in various cities around the United States, it was concluded that from 5% to 15% of the normal, presumably healthy adult population will have serious abnormalities in their exercise electrocardiograms which are indicative of the presence of severe coronary artery disease. In several of these studies, these individuals were found to be "healthy" following a standard physical examination, including a resting electrocardiogram, and their disease was diagnosed only as a result of the exercise electrocardiogram, a test which is not typically a part of a routine physical examination.

From the above, it is suggested that a comprehensive medical evaluation be undertaken prior to initiating any formal program of exercise. This obviously will be more important for those 30 years of age and older, but a sound medical evaluation is considered prudent even for the youngster who is just beginning to participate in competitive sports, whether it be Pop Warner Football, Little League Baseball, or junior high school gymnastics. An annual or semi-annual medical evaluation is considered to be a wise investment as a part of a comprehensive program of preventive medicine; thus, a clearance to participate in either sport or fitness activities could be included as a part of this examination at little or no extra cost.

COMPREHENSIVE MEDICAL EVALUATION

The standard medical examination provided today varies considerably, from a cursory 5-minute assessment of height, weight, blood pressure, and chest sounds, to a comprehensive, multi-phasic evaluation which takes several days to complete. What constitutes an appropriate medical evaluation for clearing individuals for participation in sport or exercise programs? The answer to this question depends entirely on the age of the individual and the activity or sport for which that individual is seeking clearance. The scholastic, collegiate, or professional athlete who is seeking clearance to play football will have a totally different evaluation from the middle-aged adult who is seeking clearance to join the local health club, or who wants to start a jogging program.

The Athletic Evaluation

The evaluation for clearing athletes into various sports, while concerned with the general health of the individual, includes as the major component a thorough orthopedic evaluation to identify existing injuries to bones, muscles, ligaments, tendons, and joints, and to evaluate the potential for injury. As an example, a young athlete who is diagnosed as having instability of both knees should be directed out of a high-risk contact sport such as football and encouraged to participate in a non-weight-bearing activity such as swimming or bicycling. Also included in the evaluation of athletes would be a thorough screening for cardiovascular and hematological problems. In the past several years, a number of young and apparently healthy athletes have died either during or following a particularly hard practice or a game. Cardiac arrythmias (irregular heartbeats), myocarditis (infection in the heart muscle), mitral valve prolapse (failure of the mitral valve, allowing blood to flow back into the left atrium on contraction of the left ventricle), congenital heart disease, rheumatic fever, myocardial infarction (heart attack), and sickle-cell anemia have all been implicated as primary causes of death. Most of these problems are diagnosible; thus, the appropriate cardiovascular screening procedures are essential. Finally, the athletic evaluation should include routine screening of the ears, eyes, urine, and blood. X rays are desirable, but very expensive. They may be required for certain examinations, but only recommended for others.

Before leaving this area of athletic evaluations, it is important to recognize that there are a number of physiological changes with endurance training which mimic serious medical problems. One of the classic alterations with endurance training is a substantial reduction in the resting heart rate. Many physicians are greatly concerned when they identify resting heart rates below 60 beats per minute. This is frequently diagnosed as *bradycardia,* which refers to an abnormal slow pulse or heartbeat which is the result of disease. Obviously, in the highly trained endurance athlete, this is a normal response to training and is associated with an elevated stroke volume, thus allowing for a normal cardiac output. Endurance-trained athletes have resting heart rates which are typically below 40 beats per minute, with certain individuals dropping to levels of 30 beats per minute or lower. These unusually low heart rates will frequently lead to arrythmias, where the athlete will sense an early or a late beat, or an extra or a skipped beat. At very slow heart rates, the heart is very susceptible to other areas of the heart taking over the pacemaker activity, since myocardial tissue has its own natural rate of contraction, totally independent of autonomic nervous system control.

Closely related to the above, many athletes have resting electrocardiograms which are indicative of serious heart diseases. It has only been within the past 5 to 10 years that the medical community has come to recognize these apparent abnormal electrocardiograms as normal in the highly trained athlete. For years, athletes were either sidelined or misdiagnosed as having serious heart disease. Now it is an accepted fact that these traditional abnormalities are normal variations for this highly select population of athletes. The "athlete's heart" is also another misclassification as an abnormal heart condition. Electrocardiograms and X rays indicated an enlarged left ventricle in a number of endurance-trained athletes, which in the untrained, non-athlete is a definite indication of heart disease and abnormal heart function. It is now recognized that the increase in the wall thickness of the left ventricle is a normal response to both endurance and burst-type activity. This increase in wall thickness allows for a more forceful contraction of the heart, enhancing stroke volume.

Another area in which a medical problem is diagnosed, when, in fact, the "problem" is a normal response to chronic endurance training, is the low hematocrit, which is typically associated with anemia. While the hematocrit (ratio of the red blood cells to the total blood volume) is typically low in endurance-trained athletes, either approaching or below values considered indicative of anemia in the normal individual, these athletes will have a total hemoglobin and total number of red blood cells above normal. Anemia is defined as a deficiency in either quantity or quality of blood, with the reduced quality of blood being reflected by either or both a decrease in hemoglobin levels or red blood cells. In the case of the endurance-trained athlete, the quantity as well as the quality of blood are well above normal values. The greatly increased plasma volume, however, is expanded to a much greater degree, a liter or more, than the increases in red blood cells and hemoglobin; thus, it appears as if the athlete is anemic, when, in fact, he has above-average hemoglobin and red blood cells, which are simply diluted by a greater increase in the fluid portion of the blood.

The above represent only a few of the more common problems where athletes have been misdiagnosed as having a serious disease or a clinical abnormality. In some cases, the failure to recognize the true significance of these apparent problems has resulted in the athlete being disqualified for further competition. A good general rule to follow if a significant medical abnormality is diagnosed is to get a second or third opinion by a physician or physicians who are experienced in working with athletes. Further diagnostic tests can also be administered, in some cases, to determine if there is a significant medical problem that would expose the athlete to a high risk.

The Fitness Evaluation

The medical evaluation for clearance into physical fitness programs, as was mentioned earlier, has a totally different focus from the athletic evaluation, although there are many similarities between the two. Typically, the medical evaluation for clearing participants into physical fitness programs is conducted on adults, and, thus, the identification of existing cardiovascular disease, or the risk for subsequent cardiovascular disease, becomes a dominant factor.

What should be included in a standard medical evaluation designed to clear a middle-aged adult into a comprehensive exercise program? First, it is important that the individual's physician have a comprehensive medical history, including the individual's family, as well as his personal, medical history. The family history should include incidence of heart disease, stroke, seizures, and disorders of equilibrium in close relatives, with an accurate cause and age at death. The individual's personal medical history should include any history of cardiovascular disease, including myocardial infarction, angina pectoris, undiagnosed chest pain, hypertension, rheumatic fever, murmurs, and the presence of any factors which place the individual at increased risk for coronary disease; fainting; seizures; or unstable gait. Present medication and treatment, eating habits and diet analysis, smoking history, history of alcohol intake, and the present patterns of physical activity should also be noted, along with existing athletic injuries and orthopedic problems.

Once the medical history has been obtained, the physician can start the physical examination, using the medical history to guide him in pinpointing potential problem areas. A family history of heart disease, coupled with the symptom or complaint of chest pains on exertion, leads the physician to suspect underlying coronary artery disease, and his physical examination and diagnostic tests will be oriented in that direction. The physical examination should include an investigation of bone and joint abnormalities, heart murmurs, cardiac arrythmias, abnormalities in the resting electrocardiogram, blood pressure, the presence of pulmonary emphysema or other chronic lung diseases, and the pulses in both lower extremities.

Other diagnostic tests are highly desirable in order to more completely evaluate the individual's risk for coronary artery disease. A simple blood test can provide information on blood glucose levels (elevated blood glucose levels lead to the suspicion of diabetes, a significant risk factor for coronary artery disease); total cholesterol levels and the levels of high density lipoprotein cholesterol; triglyceride levels; and uric acid levels. In addition, it is strongly suggested that anyone who is considered to have a substantial risk for coronary artery disease, or any individual 35 to 40 years of age and over, should have an exercise electrocardiogram. Table 6 (page 66) provides a greatly simplified procedure for estimating one's level of risk for each of the recognized coronary artery disease risk factors. It should be emphasized that this is strictly a guide, and it is based on the best evidence available at this time. It is also important to recognize that there would not be unanimous agreement among the scientific community relative to the validity of such a risk evaluation.

The exercise electrocardiogram has become an extremely important diagnostic tool. It was mentioned in the introduction to this chapter that in a normal population who are presumed to be healthy, and have normal resting electrocardiograms, a small but significant number of these individuals will exhibit changes in their electrocardiogram with exercise, which is indicative or suggestive of the presence of coronary artery disease. The estimates vary between 5% and 15%, depending on the sex and age of the individual. It is obviously important to identify those who have these abnormalities, for they can then be referred for further diagnostic evaluation. In some cases, these abnormal responses of the electrocardiogram during exercise are not good predictors of the presence of the disease. These are termed "false positives" on the basis of an abnormal exercise electrocardiogram, but with normal coronary arteries when the individual undergoes a catheterization procedure where a small

TABLE 6. Possible risk of the premature development of coronary artery disease

| | LEVEL OF RISK | | | | |
	VERY LOW	LOW	AVERAGE	MODERATE	HIGH
Primary Risk Factors					
Blood Pressure, mmHg					
Systolic pressure	<110	110–120	121–140	141–160	>160
Diastolic pressure	<60	60–70	71–90	91–105	>105
Cigarettes, per day	none	none	<10	11–30	>30
Blood Lipids, mg/100 ml					
Cholesterol					
Total	<180	180–195	196–220	221–260	>260
HDL, males	>64	55–64	45–54	25–44	<25
females	>74	65–74	55–64	35–54	<35
Triglycerides	<80	80–105	106–145	146–190	>190
Secondary Risk Factors					
Glucose, mg/100 ml	<80	80–95	96–115	116–135	>135
Body fat, %					
males	<10	10–14	15–20	21–26	>26
females	<15	16–20	21–26	27–33	>33
Stress-tension (subjective)	low	average	moderate	high	very high
Physical activity,* minutes	>120	60–120	15–59	<15	none
Exercise Electrocardiogram	normal	normal	normal	possibly abnormal	abnormal
Family History**	0	0	1	2	>2
Age	<31	31–40	41–50	51–60	>60
Sex		female		male	

*Minutes per week exercising at a heart rate in excess of a target rate established by subtracting your age from 220 and multiplying 0.75 {(220 − age) × 0.75} to be sustained for a minimum of 10 minutes each exercise bout
**Number of blood relatives who had heart attacks prior to age 60 years

plastic tube (catheter) is inserted into a vessel in the arm or leg and threaded up into the heart, where an opaque dye is injected into the coronary arteries. A fluoroscope is used to watch the dye travel through the coronary arteries, allowing direct visualization of any portion of the major arteries where there is significant narrowing due to the presence of coronary artery disease. The number of false positives, however, is relatively small. Therefore, there is strong support for the use of the exercise electrocardiogram both as a screening test for clearing individuals for participation in exercise programs, and as a diagnostic test to evaluate for the presence or absence of coronary artery disease.

One of the major issues in the area of exercise prescription today is whether an exercise electrocardiogram should be mandatory prior to prescribing an exercise program for an otherwise healthy person. Several years ago, there was a large segment of the medical community that felt that an exercise test was necessary, and it was then the recommendation of several major medical groups that an exercise electrocardiogram be included as a part of the medical evaluation of individuals over 35 years of age for appropriate clearance into an exercise program. While this is a sound and medically justifiable position, it is not very practical. First, most people living in rural communities have little or no access to such a screening test. Even in many larger cities, it is virtually impossible to make an appointment for an exercise electrocardiogram due to the fact that the physician conducting these tests will accept only those with known or suspected coronary artery disease. The time, facilities, equipment, and personnel are simply not sufficient to test all of those individuals who might want to start an exercise program. The second problem relates to the cost of such a test. In most communities, it will cost between $100 and $200 for the exercise test alone. This automatically takes the test out of the realm of possibility for those in the low socioeconomic sphere of society. At this point in time, most insurance companies will not pay any part of the costs of this test, unless the person is a referral for suspected coronary artery disease. Lastly, the test yields relatively few individuals who have significant coronary artery disease which had not been previously detected. It is unknown, at this time, how great a risk exercise would impose on these individuals had they been prescribed an exercise program without the benefit of an exercise electrocardiogram. At this time, the best advice appears to be to take the test if it is available and affordable, but to not be overly concerned if it isn't possible to take the test for whatever reason. It would seem that one would be at a substantially higher risk remaining sedentary because of his inability to take an exercise electrocardiogram test than to proceed with an exercise program, starting at a very low level and increasing the intensity and duration of activity at a slow rate of progression.

CONTRAINDICATIONS TO EXERCISE

There are certain medical problems which, when present, are direct contraindications to exercise. Under no circumstances are individuals to exercise when they have congestive heart failure, a recent heart attack within the past 3 months, severe anemia, myocarditis, ventricular aneurysm, uncontrolled diabetes, moderate to severe valvular disease, changing patterns of angina pectoris, and certain cardiac arrythmias. There are other medical conditions in which the individual is allowed to exercise, but only under strict medical supervision. Individuals who are likely candidates for medically supervised programs include those who have stable angina pectoris, accelerated hypertension or blood pressures greater than 180 mmHg systolic and/or 100 mm diastolic, cardiomegaly (enlarged heart), arthritis with activity, heart attack after 3 to 6 months, atrial fibrillation when under control, corrected anemia, and those patients who are under specific drug therapy.

Whenever a minor illness, injury, or infection may be aggravated by exercise, the exercise program should be terminated for an appropriate period of time. The presence of a virus always leads to the possibility of myocarditis and sudden death, even in a person with perfectly normal coronary arteries and a high level of fitness. With colds or flu, it is best to stop vigorous exercise altogether until the individual has fully recovered. Abnormal heart rhythms during exercise should be an absolute warning to stop exercising immediately!

One additional area will be mentioned, but with the realization that the information presented will usually fall on deaf ears. Once a major, or even minor, injury has been sustained, it is important in most instances to reduce the level of activity or stop activity altogether until the injury has had the appropriate time to heal. For serious athletes, or even recreational athletes or individuals who are exercising for health-related purposes, one of the most difficult things to do is to reduce the level of activity or to stop the activity altogether. As was mentioned in a previous chapter, exercise can be addictive, and if you deprive individuals of their daily dose of exercise, they actually develop withdrawal-like symptoms. Typically, these individuals refuse to adhere to sound medical advice and end up with a much more serious injury. When injured, that specific area which has been injured must have rest for a sufficient period of time during which healing can take place. Further aggravation of the injury by attempting to train through the injury usually greatly prolongs the time necessary to achieve full recovery. If the individual must have some form of activity during the period of convalescence, there are typically substitute activities that can be recommended which allow appropriate activity, but which protect the injured area. As an example, when a distance runner sustains a major knee or ankle injury, it would be foolish and medically unsound to continue with the running program until that time when sufficient healing had taken place. A good substitute activity might be pedaling a stationary bicycle, swimming, or jogging in the pool with the body submerged to the base of the neck. These activities would have to be evaluated very carefully to ensure that they were not aggravating the original injury.

One fear with any injury is the loss of physical conditioning and physiological function that accompanies the period of inactivity. Physical deconditioning occurs at a rate which is nearly a mirror image of the rate of conditioning, i.e., the benefits are lost at the same rate they were gained. It is therefore imperative for the athletic population to devise methods to maintain or at least minimize the loss of general fitness, including strength, power, muscular endurance, and cardiovascular endurance. A good physical therapist or athletic trainer who is accustomed to working with athletic injuries can usually provide the appropriate program to achieve the desired results during the period of convalescence.

PHYSICAL PERFORMANCE PROFILE

It is quite typical for the average middle-aged adult to go to his family physician for an annual or semi-annual medical evaluation with the expectation that his physician will find something wrong and be able to prescribe some form of medication which will give him an instant cure, and will provide him with unlimited energy, deep quality sleep, and a positive outlook toward life. All too often, these individuals are only disappointed when the doctor tells them that they are in perfectly good health, with no diagnosible disease. They may be a "little overweight" and probably smoke too much, but otherwise they are pronounced healthy. Most of these people are disappointed in learning what would normally be considered good news, and some will go to another doctor to seek an additional opinion. The majority of our adult American population falls into this category, where the person realizes he is not feeling well, or certainly not as well as he should, yet the physician is unable to identify any specific disease state or medical abnormality. Dr. Robert Kerlan, a highly respected sports medicine physician in Southern California, has captured the essence of this apparent paradox. According to Dr. Kerlan, the standard medical evaluation is oriented toward the detection of disease, with the patient receiving a final rating which ranges from a "0" to a "−100," "0" indicating the total absence of detectable disease, and a "−100" indicating death. A person with high blood pressure might rate a "−20," a person with controlled diabetes a "−50," and a person who had just suffered a major heart attack as a "−80." Again, the rating of "0" would include the majority of the adult American population. Dr. Kerlan has proposed that it is also possible to rate the individual on an expansion or extension of the medical evaluation scale. The ratings would be extended to include the range from "0" to a "+100," with "0" referring again to the total absence of disease, and "+100" indicating perfect health. This expanded portion of the scale from "0" to "+100" is referred to as the health evaluation, and would include an investigation into the dietary habits of the individual, his sleep patterns, smoking and alcohol intake history, his ability to cope with stress and anxiety, his emotional and spiritual stability, his patterns of physical activity, and a physical performance profile. Several of the components of the health evaluation are also major components of the medical evaluation. In fact, the physical performance profile is the unique feature of this health evaluation, for most good medical histories will provide the appropriate information in each of the other areas.

What constitutes the physical performance profile? This is a relative new concept, so it must be stated that the development of the physical performance profile is in its infancy, and the present battery of tests is being continuously modified and expanded as new information and ideas become available. Basically, most performance profiles evaluate the individual in the areas of flexibility, strength and muscular endurance, body composition (relative and absolute body fat), and cardiorespiratory endurance. Flexibility tests identify those individuals who have poor flexibility, and are at risk for chronic low back problems or other orthopedic types of complications (Figure 15, below). Strength and muscular endurance can be assessed in any one of a number of ways, using highly sophisticated and elaborate research equipment, or by simply seeing how much weight the individual can lift in a single attempt (strength), which is referred to as the one-repetition maximum, or the number of times the individual can lift a constant weight (endurance). Figure 16 (page 71) illustrates one of the newer pieces of equipment which is now being used in many research and clinical settings to measure muscular strength, power, and endurance. Body composition is assessed either by the underwater weighing technique or by estimating the body composition from diameters, circumferences, or skinfolds. These techniques were discussed in Chapter 1. Finally, the test of cardiorespiratory endurance provides the most significant information relative to this major health-related component of physical fitness. While each of the

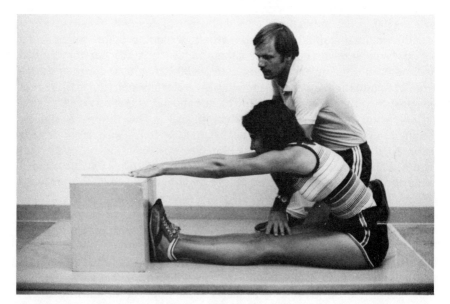

FIGURE 15. Testing the flexibility of the hamstrings muscle group and the lower back

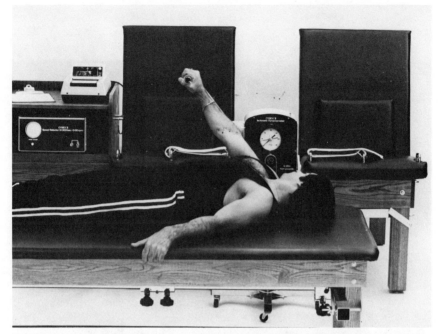

FIGURE 16. The Cybex II strength testing device, which allows an accurate assessment of strength at each point in the full range of joint movement (Photo courtesy of David Hillery, Lumex, Inc., 100 Spence Street, Bay Shore, New York 11706)

other tests is very important and provides useful information relative to the total health profile of the individual, cardiorespiratory endurance capacity is considered the basic foundation of physical fitness. The best measure of cardiorespiratory endurance capacity is the maximal oxygen uptake, measured while the person walks, jogs, or runs on the treadmill to the point of exhaustion (Figure 17, page 72). Maximal oxygen uptake values for average untrained individuals and for highly trained athletes are presented in Table 7 (page 73).

The person who had stayed in excellent physical condition through a regular exercise program will achieve a very high rating on this physical performance profile. If he also had good dietary habits, didn't smoke, consumed alcohol in moderation, got sufficient sleep, effectively coped with stress, and was emotionally and spiritually stable, this individual would rate close to the level of "+100" on the health evaluation, and would experience the feeling of optimal health and all of its associated benefits. Unfortunately, most people fall far short of optimal health. It is also highly unfortunate that many of these people believe that the way they feel is very normal for someone their age, and never attempt to improve their health profile. The health evaluation provides the person

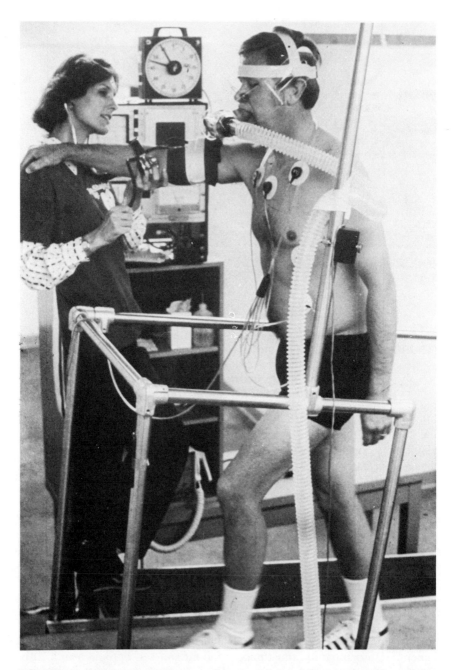

FIGURE 17. This individual is performing a treadmill test to the point of exhaustion, during which time his electrocardiogram, blood pressure, and oxygen uptake are being monitored.

TABLE 7. Maximal oxygen uptake values for normal males and females, as well as male and female athletes

GROUP	AGE	MAXIMAL OXYGEN UPTAKE, ML/KG • MIN	
		MALES	FEMALES
Untrained	10–19	47–56	38–46
	20–29	43–52	33–42
	30–39	39–48	30–38
	40–49	36–44	26–35
	50–59	34–41	24–33
	60–69	31–38	22–30
	70–79	28–35	20–27
Baseball	18–32	48–56	–
Basketball	18–30	40–55	40–44
Bicycling	18–26	62–72	47–54
Canoeing	22–28	55–67	–
Football	20–36	42–60	–
Gymnastics	18–22	52–58	34–39
Ice Hockey	10–30	50–63	–
Jockey	20–40	50–60	–
Orienteering	20–60	47–53	–
Skiing: Alpine	18–30	57–68	–
Cross-Country	20–28	65–95	60–75
Ski-Jumping	18–24	58–63	–
Soccer	22–28	54–64	–
Speed Skating	18–24	56–73	44–50
Swimming	10–25	50–70	40–55
Track and Field			
Runners	18–39	60–85	50–75
	40–75	40–60	–
Discus	22–30	42–55	–
Shot Put	22–30	40–46	–
Volleyball	18–22	–	40–47
Weightlifting	20–30	38–52	–
Wrestling	20–30	52–65	–

with objective information relative to where he is presently, and where he could be with a few changes in life-style. Individuals who have been involved in health evaluations are usually amazed when they review their results and find that there is considerable room for improvement. Even more impressive are the positive changes that occur in these individuals once they make the commitment to alter their life-styles and start to see the results of their efforts. It is not unusual to find individuals who at age 50 or 60 years are able to achieve a higher state of fitness and health than that which they had when they were young, and supposedly in the prime of their lives. Figure 18 (page 74) demonstrates this phenomenon scientifically. This is referred to as a "bad news-good news" illustration.

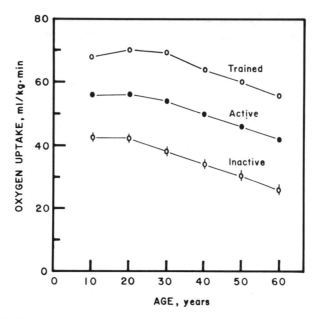

FIGURE 18. Maximal oxygen uptake in highly trained, active, and inactive individuals with aging

It is a fact of life that the maximal oxygen uptake decreases with aging, no matter whether one is sedentary, moderately trained, or highly trained. The bad news is that aging is inevitable. However, the good news is that the person who achieves a moderate state of conditioning at age 50 or 60 years will soon have the physiological capacity of the sedentary 20-year-old! That is truly good news, and may be the eternal fountain of youth which has eluded man for centuries.

4

Developing a Comprehensive Exercise Program

INTRODUCTION

Over the past decade, the science of exercise prescription has evolved, and has provided a major impetus in getting many previously sedentary individuals back on their feet and into exercise programs which are specifically designed around their likes and dislikes, their abilities and disabilities, their present state of fitness, and to provide them with the optimal dosage so they can achieve the desired benefits. Most individual exercise programs are self-designed, *i.e.,* the activity is selected and the person begins exercising. This is a potentially dangerous practice, since most people do not recognize their limitations and are likely to exceed a safe level of exercise. Just as important, people are likely to initiate an activity program without first obtaining the appropriate medical evaluation and clearance. It is highly possible that some people develop symptoms of cardiovascular disease, such as angina pectoris, make a self-diagnosis, and with a fear of their physician confirming their suspicions, they embark on their own exercise program in an attempt to correct the situation. Group programs have associated problems. Although a medical examination may be a prerequisite for participation in these programs, the exercise is typically prescribed on a mass basis and little or no attention is given to individual differences, since everyone is expected to do exactly the same thing. The individualized prescription of exercise avoids these hazards. The participant receives the appropriate medical clearance, as was discussed in the previous chapter, and his interests and physiologic capacity are individually determined, thus ensuring accurate prescription of an appropriate exercise regimen.

THE EXERCISE PRESCRIPTION

Once the individual has received medical clearance to participate in an exercise program, he can then be provided with an exercise prescription using the information from the medical and health evaluations, and the physical performance profile in particular, as the basis for this prescription. When prescribing programs of activity, attention must be given to the type or types of exercises or activities recommended, the frequency of participation, the duration of each training session and the duration of the total program, the intensity of effort, and the initial level of fitness. Each of these will be discussed briefly.

Type of Training Activity

A comprehensive exercise program will focus on more than one area of development; thus, most programs include a variety of activities. The foundation of any program, however, must be the cardiorespiratory endurance training activities. This is even true for the athlete who is training for a sport or event which may not involve cardiorespiratory endurance as a major component. Golfers, football players, baseball players, and weightlifters have little need for cardiorespiratory endurance in their specific sport or event, but these athletes as well as athletes in all sports are beginning to discover that a sound cardiorespiratory endurance foundation provides the framework from which they can more effectively develop and execute their skills. For the middle-aged adult who is seeking better health, the need for activities of a cardiorespiratory endurance nature is obvious.

Which activities are appropriate for developing cardiorespiratory endurance? While this will be discussed in substantially more detail in Chapter 6, it is appropriate to discuss the major activities at this time. The appropriate activities would be those which maintain the heart rate at its target level for a period of not less than 10 to 15 minutes. Thus, brisk walking, jogging and running, hiking, swimming, bicycling, and selected individual or dual sports such as handball, racketball, and tennis, when played vigorously, will all promote improvements in cardiorespiratory endurance capacity. Studies have been conducted which indicate that bicycling and brisk walking provide the same benefits as jogging. Other studies have shown that tennis and racketball provide improvements, but not to the same extent that you would find with jogging. The fact that the magnitude or extent of improvement wasn't as great with the sport-type activities may not be so important. First, improvement was noted, and over a period of years it is quite possible that continued participation in these activities will bring the individual up to an acceptable level of fitness.

It is appropriate at this time to differentiate between conditioning activities and maintenance activities, although the following concept is awaiting confirmation through research. A conditioning activity is one which is known to provide optimal benefits in a specific area, such as jogging in the area of cardiorespiratory endurance, and weightlifting in the area of strength and muscular endurance. A maintenance activity is one which will maintain the level of improvement achieved through the conditioning activity, and may even contribute to further development of that specific area, but is not considered a primary conditioning activity. In the area of cardiorespiratory endurance, jogging, bicycling, or swimming may be selected as the conditioning activities to increase the individual's capacity from a very low to an above-average level. Tennis, racketball, or handball may then be selected as enjoyable activities which can be undertaken to maintain, and possibly even continue to improve, the individual's level of fitness.

The concept of differentiating between conditioning and maintenance activities is an attractive one for several reasons. First, it is the feeling of many experts in the exercise and sport sciences that one should get into condition to play a sport, not play a sport to get into condition. While certain sports can be used as conditioning activities, they serve far better as maintenance activities. It is difficult to become proficient in a sport unless one is properly conditioned prior to undertaking the sport. Likewise, it is difficult to improve physical fitness through participation in a sport when the individual is not proficient in a sport. Second, conditioning activities are very boring to most individuals. Unfortunately, jogging or running has been consistently used as a form of punishment in the educational setting. Those late to a physical education class, or who were caught doing something they weren't supposed to be doing, were punished by being forced to run a lap or two around the track. It is difficult for most people to reconcile the basic inconsistency between jogging as a form of punishment on the one hand, and jogging as an enjoyable and healthy activity. If jogging were so enjoyable and beneficial, why didn't the rest of the class go out running and make those who were being punished stay back inside the building? Since many individuals simply don't enjoy conditioning activities, and will be early dropouts if they do begin a program which is strictly oriented toward conditioning activities, it has been suggested that conditioning activities be used for only the initial phase of the program. Once the individual has achieved a pre-set goal for a desirable level of cardiorespiratory endurance, that individual can then switch to a maintenance activity, which may be more enjoyable and may have a better chance of being pursued throughout that individual's lifetime. Exercise must be a lifetime pursuit. It is not possible for an individual to exercise vigorously for 2 or 3 years, then live on the residual benefits for the rest of his life. The physiological and health benefits gained are lost rapidly if the exercise program is discontinued. Therefore, it is important to have people participating in activities which they enjoy and will continue to pursue the rest of their lives.

In addition to cardiorespiratory endurance training activities, the individual may also elect to engage in stretching exercises to correct an existing problem of poor flexibility, or in strength training exercises to increase his basic level of strength and muscular endurance. These types of activities are appropriate to use in the warm-up or cool-down phase of the cardiorespiratory endurance training program. Simple static stretching and limited-strength training exercises are excellent when used prior to or immediately following the endurance workout, but a major strength training effort should be carried out on a separate day.

Frequency of Participation

With respect to frequency of participation—*i.e.,* the number of days per week that one performs his exercise program—it would appear that 3 to 4 days per week represent an optimal frequency. In this case, optimal is used to indicate the greatest return relative to the amount of time invested. Obviously, the highly skilled athlete in training for world-class competition needs to be engaged in formal training 6 to 7 days per week. For the middle-aged adult who is participating in the exercise program for its health-related benefits, it would appear that training more than 3 to 4 days per week would provide additional benefits, but the returns diminish once 3 to 4 days per week are exceeded. Several studies have shown that limited benefits may be derived from as little as 2 days per week, but this low frequency is not encouraged.

There is a tendency for individuals who have been sedentary for years, who finally make the decision to start an exercise program, to be overly motivated during the first few weeks of the program. They assume that if 3 to 4 days per week is good for them, then 6 to 7 days a week must be even better. It is far better to restrict frequency to 3 to 4 days per week at least for the first month or two, for the risk of injury or serious orthopedic complications is greatest during this initial start-up period, and the over-enthusiastic beginner may be doing far more harm than good by increasing the frequency. After the first few months of the program when the exercise habit has been firmly established and the potential for injury is reduced, it is safe to increase the frequency to 5 or 6 days per week. If exercise is being used for purposes of weight control, these additional days of exercise will facilitate the loss of body fat.

Duration of the Training Session

While several studies have indicated that cardiorespiratory endurance capacity can be improved with endurance training programs as brief as 5 to 10 minutes in duration, most research indicates that 20 to 40 minutes per day of endurance training is the optimal amount, again using optimal in the context as defined in the previous section. It must be understood that the 20 to 40 minutes represents the time invested in the cardiorespiratory endurance conditioning activities, and does not include the initial warm-up phase or the final cool-down phase.

Recent theories on the positive addiction of certain physical activities, such as jogging or distance running, suggest that exercise must be carried out for at least 30 to 40 minutes before one receives the "runner's high" and becomes positively addicted to the activity. As yet, this concept has not been scientifically validated, but discussions with those involved in running programs would tend to support these theories.

Relative to the duration of the total training program, the individual will demonstrate his greatest improvements during the first 6 months of the program. Beyond the initial 6 months, progress will still be seen, but the rate of progress will tend to diminish. Eventually, the individual will reach the point where there will be little if any further progress unless marked increases are made in either frequency, duration, or in the intensity of effort. There is no reason to encourage further progress once the desired fitness levels have been achieved, so the decision to seek further improvement, or to maintain the present level of fitness, is up to the individual. Even with the desire to continue to improve, the individual must realize that he will eventually reach his genetically determined upper level, and that further progress is impossible, even if that individual were to train 8 hours per day, 7 days per week. It is important to understand this since many individuals are highly motivated by the improvement they see in the first 6 to 12 months of their exercise program. Many who are on running programs measure their success by how much faster they are able to cover a fixed distance. They become slaves to their stopwatch, and once they reach that point where they can't run any faster, they lose interest in what they are doing and stop exercising altogether. While progress and improvement are important motivators, one must be careful not to depend too much on these factors and must learn to gain motivation from the activity itself.

Intensity of Performance

One of the most frequently asked questions by individuals who are just beginning an exercise program is: "How hard do I have to push myself?" This is also the most important question, since exercising at too high an intensity leaves one totally exhausted and is potentially dangerous for the older individual who has been sedentary for a number of years. On the other hand, exercising at too low an intensity will result in little or no improvement, since there does appear to be a minimal or threshold level of intensity which must be exceeded before improvements can be realized. This minimal or threshold level appears to be somewhere around 50% of the participant's endurance capacity. Most research studies recommend that the intensity be established at between 60% and 80% of the individual's capacity. Past experience has shown that the appropriate exercise intensity is usually overestimated and exceeded, not underestimated. This is the result primarily of the ex-athlete who recalls how hard he had to work as a boy or young man to condition himself for his sport. Unfortunately, this concept carries over into his health-related exercise program. It is, therefore, important to monitor exercise intensity to protect the individual from overdoing it, yet to make sure that the level of exercise is sufficient to result in the desired changes. How can one safely monitor exercise intensity?

Many years ago, it was theorized, and subsequent research verified, that heart rate could be effectively used to monitor the intensity of exercise. This led to the use of the term target or *training heart rate* (THR). The THR is an individually determined value that defines the precise heart rate at which that individual is to train. The THR is established most accurately by having the individual perform an exercise test on the treadmill or bicycle ergometer to the point of exhaustion or volitional fatigue. This test determines the individual's maximal capacity and maximal heart rate. He is then assigned a THR which represents a fixed percentage of that capacity. A THR set at 75% of the individual's maximal heart rate represents a level of only 60% to 65% of his maximal oxygen uptake, which has been found sufficient to produce a substantial training response.

In the absence of a maximal exercise test, it is possible to provide an estimate of the training heart rate range by using the following procedure:

Training heart rate range
    Upper level: (220 — age) x 0.80
    Lower level: (220 — age) x 0.65

Example: Age 45 years

    Upper level: (220−45) x 0.80 = 175 x 0.80 = 140 beats per minute
    Lower level: (220−45) x 0.65 = 175 x 0.65 = 114 beats per minute

Since this is strictly an estimate, and may not be appropriate for any one specific individual, it is suggested that each person subjectively evaluate how stressful the exercise bout feels to him, starting at the lower level of the THR range. Each day the person may increase the intensity by 5 beats/min. if the previous day's exercise session was perceived as being relatively easy. Even when the THR has been precisely defined by a maximal exercise test, it is not unusual for two individuals to perceive this same level of exercise differently. Some can tolerate much higher intensities, approaching 85% to 90% of their capacity without perceiving the exercise as exhaustive or too strenuous, while others have difficulty maintaining the THR, which represents only 75% of their individual capacities. It is quite possible that the perception of effort, referred to as the perceived exertion, may well represent a valid training intensity.

An additional technique which has been used to prescribe exercise intensity is through the use of METS. One MET is the equivalent of the resting metabolic rate. Various activities have been classified according to how many METS are required to perform that activity. As an example, playing singles tennis is considered a 6-MET activity, *i.e.,* it requires an average metabolic rate which is six times the resting level. Singles handball is considered a 10-MET activity. The individual's maximal exercise capacity is determined and expressed relative to MET values. As an example, since the resting metabolic rate is assumed to be 3.5 ml of oxygen per kilogram of body weight per minute, a maximal oxygen uptake of 35 ml/kg•min would be equivalent to a level of 10 METS (35 ÷ 3.5). Taking 75% of the individual's capacity would yield a training level of 7.5 METS (10 METS × 0.75). That individual would then go to that table which expresses all activities according to their MET equivalents and select from those activities which will provide him with an exercise intensity of 7.5 METS (see Table 17, Chapter 8, page 169).

The training heart rate approach for monitoring exercise intensity has distinct advantages over the MET approach. First, several research studies have indicated that the heart rate, by itself, is a very good index of the actual work being performed by the heart. This is very logical since the heart is a muscle, and the faster it beats the more work it has to do, the more energy it needs to supply its demands, and the more blood it needs to supply the increased energy demands. Using the THR approach will assure the individual that the work of the heart will remain constant irrespective of the conditions in which the individual exercises. With the MET approach, the total metabolic activity of the body is held constant, while the work of the heart can vary considerably for the same metabolic activity. If an individual had been given a MET prescription of 7.5 METS, this would be the equivalent of jogging at a pace of 5 miles per hour, or 1 mile in every 12 minutes. During cool weather at sea level, this 5-mile-per-hour jog would require an acceptable level of work by the heart. However, if the weather suddenly became warm and humid, or the individual flew to Aspen, Colorado, which is at an altitude of approximately 7,000 feet, the metabolic cost of the activity would not change—*i.e.,* 7.5 METS—but it would require a considerably greater amount of work for the heart, and, in fact, might exceed the ability of the heart. Exercise intensity should be based on the work of the heart, not on the metabolic level of the whole body. When exposed to these extremes in temperature or altitude, the body simply will do less work to attain the same THR.

One additional advantage of the THR approach over the MET approach relates to the fact that the THR automatically accounts for improvement. One of the classic changes or adaptations associated with an endurance training program is the reduction in heart rate for the same level of work, or, a higher level of work is accomplished in order to attain the same heart rate. With the THR approach, the individual is theoretically having to perform more work or perform at a higher rate of work in order to achieve the same THR. Therefore, THR doesn't have to be adjusted as the individual becomes better conditioned. With the MET approach, since the metabolic load is constant, the individual's maximum capacity must be re-evaluated periodically, and the prescribed MET level altered accordingly.

Initial Fitness Level

The initial fitness level of those starting an exercise program is also an important consideration when prescribing exercise. Individuals with low endurance fitness will be started on a much more conservative program. The THR will be maintained at 70% to 75% of their maximal heart rate and the rate of progression will be slow. Individuals with high endurance fitness can be started on a program with a THR representing 80% to 85% of their maximal heart rate and can proceed at a much faster rate of progression.

THE EXERCISE PROGRAM

Once medical clearance has been obtained and the exercise prescription determined, it is necessary to integrate all of the information described above into a total exercise program. The total exercise program should include: a warm-up and stretching period; the endurance conditioning period; the cool-down period; and, if desired, a strength conditioning period.

The warm-up and stretching period is intended to serve two specific purposes. First, it is important to gradually prepare the body for the strenuous endurance conditioning period which follows. Therefore, the individual starts with low-level activity and progresses to more vigorous activity. Improvement of flexibility is a second purpose of this period. Static stretching exercises are integrated with calisthenic-type warm-up exercises to provide 5 to 15 minutes of continuous activity. A sound warm-up and stretching period will help reduce the amount of muscle and joint soreness that is typically experienced during the first few weeks of an exercise program. In addition, recent studies at U.C.L.A. have found that individuals who proceed directly into vigorous exercise without prior warm-up will demonstrate serious abnormalities in their electrocardiogram during the first few seconds of this activity. Appropriate warm-up, stretching, and cool-down exercises will be discussed in much greater detail in the next chapter.

The endurance conditioning period is the "heart" of the total exercise program. The exercise prescription, described in the preceding section, outlines all of the details of this period. Once the type of activity has been selected, and the frequency and duration of exercise established, it is important to properly define the THR. During the initial 2 to 3 weeks of the program, the individual should stop approximately every 5 minutes in the endurance conditioning period and monitor his pulse rate. The radial artery on the thumb side of the wrist, or the carotid artery in the upper part of the neck, just to the side and slightly above the larynx, can be palpated with the fingers of the right hand. Using the second hand of a wristwatch or clock, count the number of pulses in a 15-second period, and multiply this count by 4 to derive the number of beats per minute. The pulse rate stays elevated at its exercise rate for the initial 10 to 15 seconds of the recovery period, so if the count is taken immediately upon stopping exercise, the derived pulse rate is an accurate index of the true rate during the last few minutes of exercise. If the derived rate upon stopping exercise is below the THR, then the intensity of exercise should be increased. If it is above the THR, the intensity should be decreased. After several weeks of monitoring, the individual learns to read his body and can stay very close to his THR with only periodic monitoring of the rate.

The cool-down period is extremely important, for the demands of the muscles during exercise have opened up a number of blood vessels in the active muscles. If the exercise was predominantly a lower-body exercise, such as jogging or bicycling, there would be a large volume of blood starting to pool in the veins of the lower extremities immediately upon the cessation of exercise. If the individual were just to stop exercising and stand in place, this pooling of blood could lead to nausea, dizziness, and fainting. Cool-down exercises combine stretching with active walking, or some other form of rhythmic activity, to assist the blood back to the heart through the squeezing-effect rhythmic muscle contraction has on the veins in the immediate area. This low-level activity also helps to reduce the degree of subsequent muscle soreness.

SPECIAL EXERCISE PROGRAMS

There are certain individuals who should exercise only in a structured program under the direct supervision of a physician or his designate. The medical problems which would place one in this category were outlined in the previous chapter. In general, individuals in medically monitored programs follow almost identical guidelines to those discussed above. The major difference would be in the selection of activities, in the intensity of participation, and in the rate of progression. Due to the restrictive nature of a medically supervised program having to be conducted in a relatively small area where all participants must exercise within view of the physician, nurse, or trained technician, this by necessity restricts the selection of activities available. Most medically supervised programs provide walk/jog/run activity, swimming or stationary bicycling, and equipment for upper body development. The intensity of the exercise is scaled to the nature of the medical problem. If a patient develops significant arrythmias or heart irregularities during exercise at a certain heart rate, then the THR is adjusted well below this level. Lastly, the rate of progression is very slow for most patient groups. It is far better to be conservative in approach, rather than to place the patient in a high-risk situation. There have been several notable exceptions to this conservative approach. Dr. Terrance Kavanagh of Toronto, Ontario, and Dr. Jack Scaff of Honolulu, Hawaii, both practicing cardiologists, have trained selected post-coronary patients to run in full 26.2-mile marathons. Not all heart attack victims can be trained to this level, nor should they try, but this does point to the degree of recovery some of these patients can attain.

Unfortunately, not every community has a physician-supervised exercise program available to those patients who should be in such programs. What does the patient do? Exercise is considered to be an essential part of the therapy in the rehabilitation of most of the diseases which are assigned to this category of physician-supervised program. Is the patient safer to remain sedentary and lose the positive benefits of the exercise program, or is it safer for him to exercise on his own recognizing the need to proceed with caution? For most patients, the latter course would be recommended, and, in fact, is the standard approach of most physicians today. If one of their patients has a heart attack, and a supervised program isn't available when the patient reaches that point in his recovery where exercise is considered important, the physician will typically send the patient off on his own, starting with very low levels of activity. Obviously, the conservative approach is called for at this point. Exercise should be at a very low intensity and the rate of progression should be very gradual. In addition, the spouse, relative, neighbor, or a close friend should be encouraged to accompany the patient during each exercise session, and should be trained in cardiopulmonary resuscitation procedures in the event of complications. The patient should also be instructed as to how he can closely monitor his body signs and symptoms. When he starts to sense that he is having difficulty, he can reduce the intensity or stop the exercise altogether and then consult with his physician to determine if it is safe for him to continue at a later date.

THE EDUCATED CONSUMER

When one finally makes the commitment to begin an exercise program, he is suddenly placed in a vulnerable position, at the mercy of those who are trying to sell equipment, books, and memberships in health clubs or fitness centers, just to name a few. The final section of this chapter will deal specifically with a few basic pointers on how to invest wisely.

One of the first decisions that has to be made concerns the location or facility where the exercise program will be conducted. Obviously, the first, and sometimes best, choice is the individual's home and/or neighborhood. Will he be able to follow a personal program of exercise in his own home or around his local neighborhood? Many joggers take this approach and it works out most satisfactorily for the majority of them. However, if the program includes weight training, or a sport such as racketball, this may well take the exercise program away from the home and into some community or commercial agency. How does one select from among all of the choices available to him? It is not unusual to have programs available through the local Y.M.C.A., Y.W.C.A., Y.M.H.A., Y.W.H.A., local public school, community or state college, university, health club or spa, fitness center, or sports center. Usually, financial considerations will, by necessity, take precedence in the final decision-making process. However, there are other considerations which need to be resolved to assure the individual that he is making the correct choice.

First, the issue of cost and specifically what is included for that cost must be clarified. Often, costs are hidden, and it is only after the final contract has been signed that the full costs are disclosed. If there are several facilities under consideration, it is wise to conduct a simple cost/benefit ratio. One facility may cost slightly more, but may provide much more in the way of equipment, space, and experienced personnel. Is the equipment available which will be needed in the individualized exercise program? Is instruction or supervision available? Will the facility be open and available at those times when the individual can use or desires to use the facility? Does the facility have an established reputation? Are the instructors and supervisors knowledgeable, and have they been trained properly, *e.g.,* undergraduate college degree in physical education? These and other questions should be answered before a final decision is made. If there is a state college or university in the local vicinity, there will usually be an exercise physiologist on the faculty who can assist the individual in making this decision. In many instances, the local state college or university will have established its own adult fitness program. These are typically sound programs with good facilities, well-trained personnel, excellent testing programs, and are usually very reasonably priced.

In 1975, The Association of Physical Fitness Centers was formed by a group of concerned physical fitness oriented companies. The association is dedicated to maintaining standards in health spa, health club, and fitness center operations. They have established a code of ethical practices which each member must adhere to to remain in good standing. The association's national office is located in Suite 500, 5272 River Road, Washington, D.C. 20016, and maintains an active file of its membership. The code of ethics was developed to protect the consumer, so a member organization in good standing represents a sound business operation.

The individual is frequently placed in the position of having to make decisions relative to clothing, shoes, and special equipment, such as rackets, clubs, and indoor exercise devices. When the exercise prescription specifies games like tennis or racketball, or an indoor exercise device such as a stationary bicycle, proper knowledge of the equipment under consideration is important. It would be impossible in this book to discuss all possible items of equipment likely to be used in an exercise program. However, there are certain guidelines that can be applied in the purchase of most specialized exercise equipment, including the following:

1. Deal with reputable businesses that will stand behind their products.
2. Consult experts in the field, or various consumer reports, if there is any question about a company or its product. Most Y.W.C.A.'s, colleges, or universities have experts in this area who would be willing to provide assistance.
3. Avoid devices that claim to do all of the work. Active participation is essential to obtain the desired benefits of exercise.
4. Do not be misled into thinking that the more expensive the item, the better job it does. Many items of equipment are greatly overpriced.
5. Do not buy something that will not be used. Many expensive items of exercise equipment end up being stored in the garage, basement, or attic.
6. Do not buy on impulse after receiving a high-powered sales pitch. Wait at least three days before making the final decision.
7. Understand completely the purpose of the exercise device and its principle of operation.

Finally, many sports have become so popular that specialized magazines have been started to cater to the specific needs and interests of participants in those sports. These magazines typically provide sound articles and information relative to consumer affairs, in addition to articles on training techniques, strategies, and other areas of interest. As an example, *Runner's World* magazine is a monthly publication for runners of both sexes, all ages, and all abilities. It devotes one issue each year

(October) to rating the various running shoes. This is an outstanding consumer service which has forced the shoe manufacturers to improve on shoe design and to produce a better-quality shoe.

In summary, the information is there if the consumers will take the time to ask the appropriate questions and to do a little homework. Literally millions of dollars are foolishly spent each year because consumers simply did not take the time to become informed. Informed consumers will make reasonable demands on the free-enterprise system, which will only work to improve the quality of products and service over a period of time.

5

The Warm-Up, Stretching, and Cool-Down Periods

INTRODUCTION

The importance of an appropriate warm-up and stretching period and a cool-down period was discussed in detail in the previous chapter. The warm-up and stretching period is designed to stretch the muscles for the purpose of increasing or maintaining proper flexibility of the major joints, and to gradually prepare the whole body for the endurance conditioning period. How important is this warm-up and stretching period? It is not unusual to see athletes bypass the warm-up and stretching period and proceed directly into the endurance conditioning phase. This is also true of many recreational joggers, who simply start jogging without the appropriate warm-up and stretching period. These individuals typically justify their actions by stating that they start slowly, using the initial part of their endurance conditioning period as the warm-up to a faster pace which follows. What does research conclude with respect to the value of warm-up and stretching?

Most research on warm-up has looked at its importance relative to athletic performance—*i.e.,* is warm-up essential in order to achieve the best athletic performance? This question is much more complex than it may appear on the surface, for there are various forms of warm-up. As an example, for the baseball player, there are specific (throwing) and general (calisthenics) activities which are considered active forms of warm-up. In addition, there are also passive forms of warm-up, such as hot showers, massage, or heating pads. With this in mind, the research would tend to indicate that warm-up facilitates accuracy, speed of movement, range of motion, and strength in movements of selected parts of the body, but it doesn't affect reaction time. Sprints and distance runs are improved with warm-up, but agility runs are not. Baseball-throwing speed and softball distance throw are improved with warm-up, but accuracy of the throw appears to be unaffected by warm-up. Most coaches and athletes feel that warm-up is essential to prevent injuries, but there is very little direct research evidence to support their beliefs. The study referred to in the previous chapter demonstrated significant abnormalities in the exercise electrocardiogram when burst-type activities were performed without prior warm-up. Even though the research literature is equivocal relative to the benefits of warm-up, it would appear prudent to include warm-up activities as an important part of the total exercise program until more substantial evidence surfaces to indicate that it could be safely omitted.

Stretching exercises are extremely beneficial in developing increased flexibility. Athletes who don't stretch are much more susceptible to musculoskeletal problems or injuries, such as sprains, strains, and muscle pulls. Certain types of endurance conditioning activities actually work to decrease an individual's flexibility! Most distance runners who ignore stretching exercises are usually able to reach their kneecaps, but not much farther, when asked to touch their toes. Running over a period of months or years will definitely reduce flexibility in the legs and lower back, and will occasionally lead to chronic lower back problems if not corrected.

Flexibility can be markedly improved in a relatively short period of time. The specific stretching exercises are very simple to perform and require relatively little time. Professor Herbert deVries of the University of Southern California has pioneered much of the work in stretching exercises to increase flexibility. He has defined two types of flexibility: static and dynamic. Static flexibility refers to the total range of motion of a particular joint, while dynamic flexibility refers to the ease with which a joint moves through it range of motion during dynamic activity. When a muscle contracts quickly or in a jerky motion, it will stretch the antagonistic muscles causing them to contract, thus reducing the range of motion. A firm static stretch involves a specific neuromuscular reflex which results in an inhibition of the antagonistic group of muscles, thus increasing the range of motion.

Flexibility can be increased through rapid or ballistic types of movements, such as bobbing or jerking, or through slow controlled stretching. Using hip flexion as an example, in the ballistic approach the individual would lean forward at the waist, keeping the knees locked out in full extension, and bounce or bob up and down, attempting to touch his toes. In controlled stretching, sometimes referred to as static stretching, the individual will lean forward, grab his ankles, and then very slowly pull himself downward, placing the muscles on slow stretch. Research has shown both methods to be equally effective, but the controlled stretching technique is advocated since there appears to be less danger of injury and soreness, and the antagonist group of muscles are fully relaxed.

THE WARM-UP AND STRETCHING PERIOD

The warm-up and stretching period can last from several minutes to 10 or 15 minutes, depending on the need for thorough warm-up and stretching. Those who have acceptable levels of flexibility, and who warm-up quickly, may need only a few minutes of stretching and light calisthenics to prepare themselves for the endurance conditioning period. Others may be slow starters, and may need to concentrate on a number of specific stretching exercises to improve their flexibility. Thus, the content of the warm-up and stretching period will be totally dependent on the needs and desires of the individual. The following exercises have been selected as appropriate for inclusion in the warm-up and stretching period. The number of repetitions for each exercise will vary from one exercise to the next, and according to the fitness level and ability of the individual. Therefore, recommendations for repetitions have been established for three different levels: A—beginning; B—intermediate; and C—advanced.

1. Head rotation

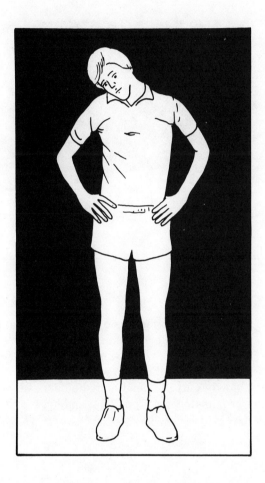

Purpose: to stretch the muscles of the neck and upper back
Start: standing upright with the hands on the hips, and the
                feet placed shoulder-width apart
Movement: slowly rotate the head clockwise in a full circle for
                the specified number of repetitions; then reverse the
                direction for an equal number of repetitions
Repetitions: A, B, and C—5

2. Head and shoulder curl

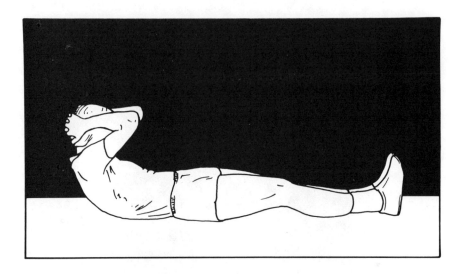

Purpose: to stretch the muscles of the neck and upper back, and to promote abdominal strength

Start: lie on the back with the legs fully extended forward, and the hands behind the head or neck

Movement: slowly curl the head and shoulders forward to approximately a 45° position, and hold for 5 seconds

Repetitions: A—4; B—6; C—8

3. Trunk rotation

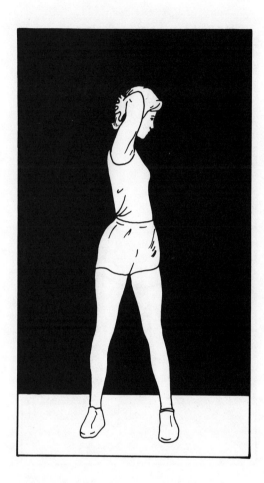

Purpose:	to stretch the muscles of the back, sides, and shoulder girdle
Start:	stand upright, hands behind the head, and the feet placed shoulder-width apart
Movement:	rotate the trunk as far to the right as possible, and then rotate as far to the left as possible
Repetitions:	A—5; B—10; C—15

4. Chest and shoulder stretch

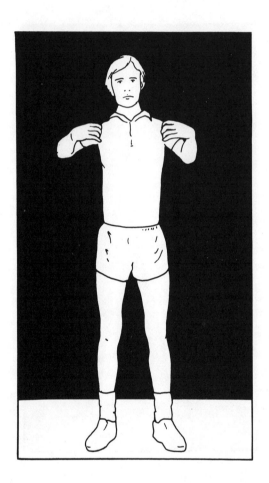

Purpose: to stretch the muscles of the chest and shoulder girdle

Start: stand upright, elbows extended outward at shoulder level, the feet placed shoulder-width apart

Movement: pull the elbows back as far as possible, holding for several seconds and return to the starting position

Repetitions: A—5; B—10; C—15

5. Bar hang

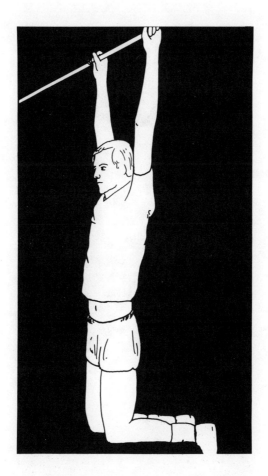

Purpose: to stretch the muscles of the arms, shoulders, back, trunk, and hips

Start: grab the bar with the palms of the hands facing forward

Movement: hang from the bar for 60 seconds

Repetitions: A, B, and C—1

6. Hip rotation

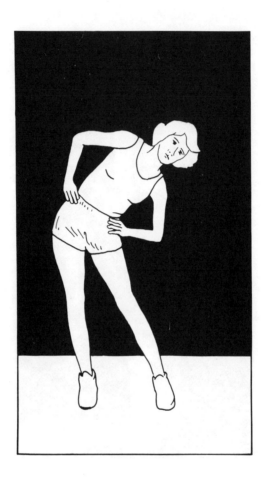

Purpose: to stretch the muscles of the hips and back
Start: stand upright, hands on hips, with the feet placed shoulder-width apart
Movement: bending at the waist, rotate the trunk to the right side, forward, left side, and return
Repetitions: A—5; B—10; C—15

7. Push-up, modified and full

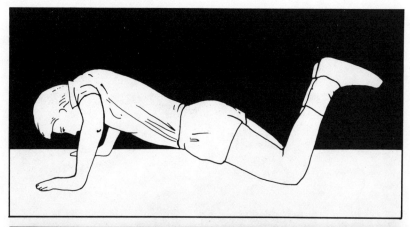

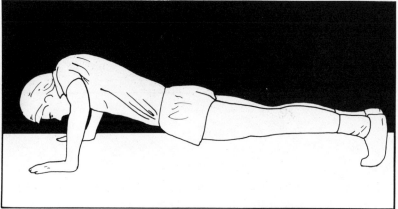

Purpose: to strengthen the muscles of the upper arm and shoulder girdle

Start: arms fully extended, shoulder-width apart supporting the upper body weight, with the feet extended backward, the toes supporting the lower body weight

Movement: slowly lower the chest to the floor, keeping the back straight and in line with the buttocks, then push back up to the fully extended position

Repetitions: A—10; B—20; C—30 or more

Note: For those with limited upper body strength, perform this exercise with the knees on the floor, forming the point of support. Move to the full push-up when 30 repetitions can be performed.

8. Back hyperextension

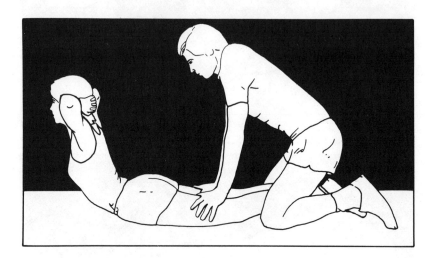

Purpose:	to stretch the abdominal and chest muscles and to strengthen the lower back
Start:	lie on the stomach, with the legs extended to the rear, and the hands behind the head.
Movement:	with a partner holding the feet, slowly extend the trunk upward as far as possible and hold for 3 to 5 seconds
Repetitions:	A—2; B—4; C—6

9. Backward single leg raise

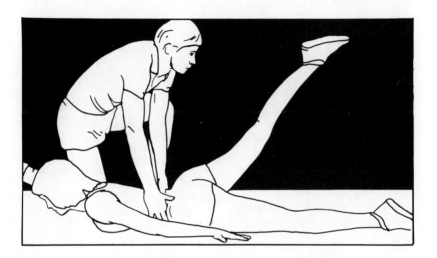

Purpose: to stretch the muscles of the hip and abdomen and to tighten the buttocks

Start: lie on the stomach with the legs extended to the rear, arms to the side

Movement: with a partner holding the hips and lower back in place, lift the right leg up as high as possible, keeping the stomach and hips pressed flat against the floor, and hold for 3 to 5 seconds; repeat with the opposite leg

Repetitions: A—2; B—4, C—6

10. Single knee to chest

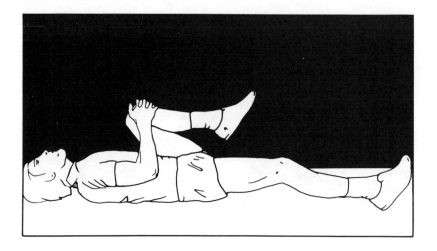

Purpose: to stretch muscles in the lower back and buttocks
Start: lie on the back with the legs extended forward
Movement: bring the right knee up and into the chest, pulling the knee with the hands and arms as far forward as possible, hold in the fully stretched position for 5 seconds, and then repeat with the opposite leg
Repetitions: A—3; B—6; C—9

11. Double knee to chest

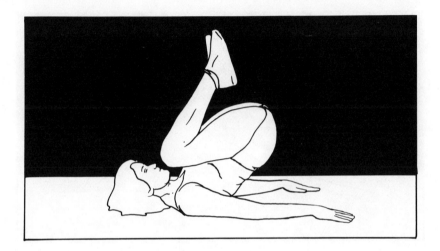

Purpose: to stretch the hamstrings and lower back muscles
Start: lie on the back with the arms to the side, and the legs extended forward
Movement: bring both knees up toward the head, keeping the arms and upper back pressed firmly against the floor, hold for 5 seconds, and then relax
Repetitions: A—3; B—6; C—9

12. Forward praying

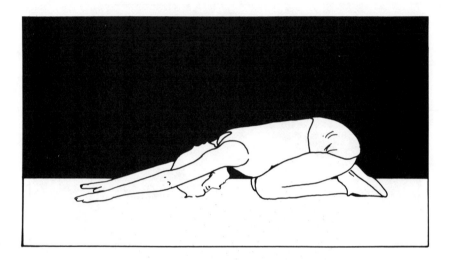

Purpose: to stretch the muscles of the lower back and hips
Start: kneel on the hands and knees, with the knees spread slightly apart and directly under the hips
Movement: keeping the hands and knees in position, lower the buttocks until it touches the heels, and extend the arms forward and lower the chest to the floor and hold for 5 seconds
Repetitions: A—3; B—6; C—9

13. Bent-knee sit-up

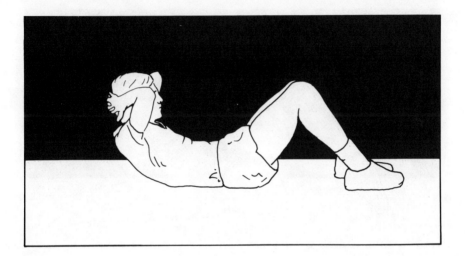

Purpose: to strengthen the abdominal and hip flexor muscles

Start: lie on the back with the knees bent to a 90° angle, and the hands clasped behind the head

Movement: curl the head, shoulders and back up to the full sitting position touching one of the knees with the opposite elbow

Repetitions: A—5; B—20; C—30 or more

14. The "Plough"

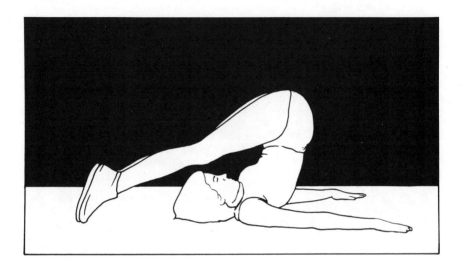

Purpose: to stretch the muscles of the lower back and hips

Start: lie on the back with the legs extended forward, and the arms extended to the side

Movement: keeping the legs locked into extension at the knees, raise the legs up and over the head, attempting to touch the floor behind the head with the toes

Repetitions: C—3

15. Kneeling back arch

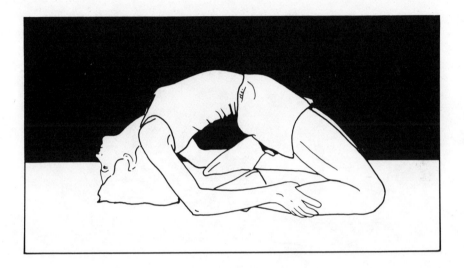

Purpose:	to stretch the abdominal and hip flexor muscles
Start:	assume an upright kneeling position with the toes pointed backward
Movement:	slowly lean backward, attempting to touch the head to the floor
Repetitions:	C—3

16. Pike position

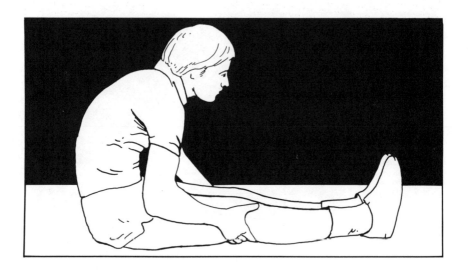

Purpose: to stretch the hamstrings and lower back muscles
Start: assume a sitting position with the legs extended forward and the knees pressed flat on the floor
Movement: grasp behind the knees and slowly pull the trunk down toward the knees, holding the stretched position for 5 seconds
Repetitions: A—4; B—6; C—8

17. Lower leg and heel stretcher

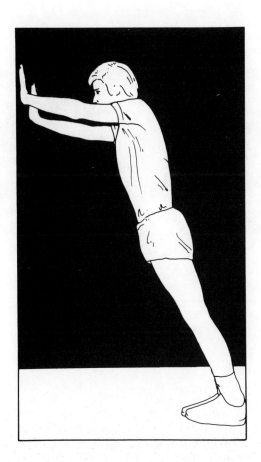

Purpose: to stretch the muscles of the lower leg and the Achilles' tendon

Start: stand upright approximately 3 feet from a wall or post

Movement: keeping the feet flat on the floor, extend the arms forward touching the wall and slowly allow the body to lean forward, holding the stretched position for 5 seconds

Repetitions: A—4; B—6; C—8

18. Groin stretcher

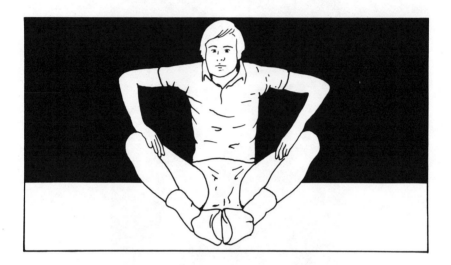

Purpose:	to stretch the groin muscles
Start:	assume a sitting position, bottoms of the feet together, and the knees pointing outward
Movement:	slowly push down on the knees, holding the stretched position for 5 seconds
Repetitions:	A—4; B—6; C—8

These 18 exercises represent only a selected few. There are many additional warm-up and stretching exercises which could be substituted for any of the above. Non-cultic Yoga provides an entire series of excellent exercises which help tone and stretch the muscles and tendons of the body. It should be re-emphasized that all stretching movements should be done slowly and carefully. Several of the above exercises are recommended only for the advanced level, since they require extreme coordination and good existing flexibility.

THE COOL-DOWN PERIOD

The purpose of the cool-down period is to assist in the return of blood to the heart by simple rhythmic contractions of those muscles used in the endurance conditioning period, and to stretch the active muscles to help relieve existing soreness and prevent future soreness. For the former, it is usually appropriate to continue or modify the endurance conditioning activity, such as walking following a jog or run, or pedaling the bicycle or swimming at a very slow rate. Just as the body is gradually prepared for the endurance conditioning period by a progressive increase in the level of activity during the warm-up and stretching period, it is important that the level of activity be gradually decreased during the cool-down period.

With respect to the stretching exercises to prevent or reduce muscle and joint soreness, specific exercises can be selected from those proposed above for the warm-up and stretching period. All exercises that are selected, however, should follow the initial phase of the cool-down period, in which the conditioning activity or a modification of the conditioning activity is performed at a reduced intensity. Also, these stretching exercises should be performed relatively close to one another in succession, so the body doesn't cool down too quickly, causing the individual to be chilled.

ASSESSMENT OF FLEXIBILITY

The most accurate tests of flexibility presently available are those tests which assess the actual range of motion of the various joints. However, the equipment necessary for such an assessment is both expensive and not readily available. Also, since flexibility is specific to each joint, no generalized flexibility test is available. However, since most of the medical problems associated with poor flexibility are related to the lower back, a simple test for assessing the flexibility of the lower back is proposed, which is referred to as the sit-and-reach test. This test is illustrated in Figure 15, Chapter 3 (page 70).

In the sit-and-reach test, the individual sits upright with his legs extended directly in front of him, his heels spread about 5 inches apart, and the knees are pressed flat against the floor. A yardstick is taped to the floor between the individual's legs with the 15-inch mark in line with the heels of the feet, the low numbers on the yardstick toward the individual. He then bends forward slowly at the waist reaching as far forward on the yardstick as possible. The score is taken as the most distant point reached on the yardstick with the fingertips fully extended. The best of three trials is then used as an index of that individual's trunk flexibility and can be compared to the norms in Table 8 (below). It is advisable to allow the individual an opportunity to have a short warm-up period of stretching exercises prior to administering the test. During the test, the movement should be one of slow stretch not fast or ballistic types of movement. Finally, this test is influenced by the length of the arms and legs, but this is a rather minor influence.

TABLE 8. Standards for the sit-and-reach flexibility test

CATEGORY	VALUE, INCHES
Excellent	22 or greater
Good	19–21
Average	14–18
Fair	12–13
Poor	11 or less

The Cardiorespiratory Endurance Period

INTRODUCTION

Cardiorespiratory endurance should be the major focus of any conditioning program. It is important to recognize that cardiorespiratory endurance is not the same as muscular endurance. Muscular endurance is a local phenomenon, and refers to the ability of the muscle or muscle group to sustain prolonged exercise. The exercise can be either of a rhythmical or repetitive nature—*e.g.,* pull-ups or push-ups—or of a static nature, such as in a sustained isometric contraction. The resulting fatigue is confined to the local group of muscles which had been exercised. Cardiorespiratory endurance is a more general, total body phenomenon, and refers to the ability of the total body to sustain prolonged rhythmical exercise. Muscular endurance is highly related to muscular strength, while cardiorespiratory endurance reflects the development and status of the cardiovascular and respiratory systems. Muscular endurance will be discussed in more detail in the following chapter.

Endurance conditioning, which will refer specifically to conditioning to develop one's cardiorespiratory endurance capacity, can be achieved in a number of ways. Probably the most popular form of endurance conditioning at the present time is jogging or long-distance running. According to the President's Council on Physical Fitness and Sports and a recent Gallup Poll, titled "American Exercise Survey," the number of adult runners grew from a handful in 1960 to 6,000,000 in 1972, 11,000,000 in 1975, and 17,000,000 in 1978. There are more than 200 marathon races each year which have been officially sanctioned as 26.2 miles in length, and over 50,000 Americans have successfully completed at least one marathon. Several marathon races in 1979 drew more than 10,000 starters!

But even with jogging or long-distance running there are variations in how one trains. There are those who advocate interval training, where short periods of rest are interspersed with periods of intense work, and there are others who advocate LSD training, which is an acronym for long slow-distance training, where the exercise is continuous but at a low intensity. The following section will discuss these and other training systems. While the discussion will be largely oriented toward walking, jogging, and running, these systems are equally effective for other forms of endurance conditioning, such as bicycling or swimming, but they are not necessarily applicable to the various sports which are used as maintenance activities, and which will be discussed in detail in Chapter 8.

TRAINING SYSTEMS

The major training systems which will be discussed will include interval training, continuous training, which includes LSD training, circuit training, and then a combination approach to training.

Interval Training

The system of interval training, which is presently very popular for training individuals ranging from world-class athletes to patients in medically supervised rehabilitation programs, has had its origins traced back to Germany in the early 1930s. This system was supposedly the result of the collaboration of a coach and a physiologist. Interval training involves the insertion of rest intervals, or, more typically, intervals of reduced activity, referred to as relief intervals, between intervals of work. Basic research in the laboratory has demonstrated that a considerably greater amount of work can be performed when the total work is broken into short, intense bouts with rest intervals interspersed between consecutive work bouts. The intervals of work and rest are usually equal, and can vary from several seconds to 5 minutes or more. In addition to the terms "work interval" and the "rest or relief interval," the vocabulary of interval training also includes the terms "set," "repetitions," "training time," "training distance," and "frequency." The term "set" describes a series of work and relief intervals. As an example, a typical set might include 8 400-meter runs at a pace of 70 seconds each, with a 60-second period of light jogging as the relief interval. "Repetitions" refer to the number of work intervals within one set. Using the above example, the number of repetitions would be 8. "Training time" refers to the rate at which the work is to be accomplished during the work interval. In the above example the training time was 70 seconds to complete each 400-meter run. "Training distance" is the distance of the work interval, or 400 meters in the above example. "Frequency" has the same meaning as has been used in previous chapters, *i.e.,* the number of training days per week.

A typical interval training prescription for a single day's workout would be as follows.

Set 1: 6 × 400 meters at 75 seconds (90 seconds jog)
Set 2: 6 × 800 meters at 180 seconds (200 seconds jog-walk)

For Set 1, the athlete would run 6 repetitions of 400 meters each, completing the work interval in 75 seconds, with a relief interval of 90 seconds of jogging. In Set 2, the individual would run 6 repetitions of 800 meters each, completing the work interval in 180 seconds, with a relief interval of 200 seconds of jogging and walking. According to Fox and Mathews in their excellent text entitled *Interval Training: Conditioning for Sports and General Fitness,* the actual stimulus for conditioning is accomplished by manipulating any one or more of the following 5 variables: 1) rate and distance of the work interval; 2) number of repetitions during each set and the number of sets per workout; 3) the duration of the rest or relief interval; 4) type of activity during the relief interval; and 5) the frequency of training per week.

The major advantage of interval training according to its proponents is the fact that you can accomplish the same amount of work and experience less fatigue. As an example, if the individual were to run as far as possible in 3 minutes on one day, and perform the same intensity of work in 3 1-minute bouts, with a 1-minute rest interval between work bouts, he would have covered the same distance in the same period of time, but the degree of fatigue would be considerably less. The major reason for the lower level of fatigue is the fact that a different source of immediate energy is being used in the interval training which results in the production of substantially lower amounts of lactic acid. Of course, the total workout time will be extended substantially by the addition of the relief or rest intervals.

One of the keys to a successful interval training program is selecting the appropriate intensity or work rate. The THR approach outlined in Chapter 4 has been commonly used to monitor work intensity. THR will be established on the basis of two variables: the maximal heart rate and the desired intensity. Maximal heart rate is best obtained during a monitored exercise test. It can also be estimated on the track in young, healthy, well-trained individuals. The person simply runs one lap around the track (440 yards) at top speed, then monitors the pulse rate during the first 15 seconds of recovery. The 15-second value multiplied by a factor of 4 will provide an estimate of the maximal heart rate in beats per minute. It will then be necessary to determine if the intervals are to be run at 95% of the maximum heart rate (high intensity), at an intensity between 80% and 95%

of maximal heart rate (moderate intensity), or at an intensity below 80% (low intensity). In some cases, the duration of the relief interval is dictated by the return of the heart rate during the relief interval to a pre-set level. Once the heart rate reaches this level, the next work interval begins. For individuals 30 years of age and younger, it is a common practice to allow the pulse rate to drop to a value between 130 and 150 beats per minute before starting the next repetition, and to 120 beats per minute before starting the next set. For those over 30 years of age, since the maximum pulse rate drops by approximately 1 beat per minute per year, it would be appropriate to reduce the above pulse rate guidelines by 1 beat per minute for each year over age 30. The 55-year-old would decrease the above guidelines by 25 beats per minute (55 years − 30 years = 25), and would use between 105 and 125 beats per minute for his recovery pulse between repetitions, and 95 beats per minute for his recovery pulse between sets. Since absolute accuracy is not critical, it is sometimes easier to take a 6-second pulse count and then multiply the resulting value by a factor of 10. This can result in an error as large as 10 beats per minute, but this is an acceptable accuracy rate for these purposes.

An easier technique can be used to determine the rate of work, and this is largely a trial-and-error technique. If the desired number of repetitions cannot be achieved at the established work rate or pace, then the pace is too fast. On the other hand, if the desired number of repetitions is completed and the individual feels he could comfortably perform additional repetitions, then the pace is too slow. In short, the individual should be at or near exhaustion by the time he reaches his last repetition.

The length of the work interval, both time and distance, will vary depending on the purpose of training. For the elite sprinter, the work intervals are typically short, 200 to 400 meters or less, while the distance runner will concentrate on work intervals that will vary between 400 meters and 1,500 meters or more. Theoretically, this type of training will allow an athlete to complete his racing distance at top speed, without experiencing fatigue or exhaustion toward the end of the run. The number of repetitions and sets will also be largely determined by the sport, activity, or event. Generally, the shorter and more intense the interval, the greater the number of repetitions and sets. Correspondingly, as the training interval is lengthened in both distance and duration, the number of repetitions and sets is reduced. Fox and Mathews have established a series of guidelines which can be followed in the selection of repetitions and sets.

The type of activity during the relief interval can vary from slow walking to rapid walking and jogging, or the equivalent in other activities. Generally, the more intense the work interval, the less intense the relief interval. With increased levels of conditioning, the intensity of the work interval can be increased, or the duration of the rest interval can be decreased.

The above concepts of interval training can be applied to many different sports or activities and should not be considered applicable only to running. In the excellent text of Fox and Mathews, referred to above, specific programs for various sports are proposed, illustrating how the interval training procedure applies to the conditioning of athletes who participate in these sports. Interval training procedures are also used in the conditioning of previously sedentary adults. However, the work intensity is scaled to their fitness level.

Continuous Training

Continuous training, as its name implies, involves continuous activity without rest intervals. This can vary from high-intensity activity of moderate duration to low-intensity activity of an extended duration. Long slow-distance (LSD) training is a classic example of the latter. High-intensity exercise is typically defined as working at intensities that represent 85% to 95% of the individual's maximal heart rate. For the distance runner, this represents a pace which is slightly below his racing pace; however, this will vary considerably depending on the distance of both the competition run and the training run. There is one major advantage of this type of training. The runner is training at a pace which closely approximates his race pace, and this helps not only in conditioning the athlete, but in helping him to regulate his pace, since running at an even pace has been proven to be the most efficient way to race and should result in the best time. Too much high-intensity training, however, should be avoided since it is extremely stressful and may lead to serious injury. Low-intensity training should be substituted periodically—*i.e.*, once or twice per week—to provide relief from this exhaustive form of training.

Low-intensity continuous training is probably the most popular form of training for those who are participating in an exercise program for its health-related benefits. It is popular because it is much less stressful than either interval training or high-intensity continuous training. LSD training became popular toward the end of the 1960s, and its origins have been traced back to Dr. Ernst VanAaken, a German physician and coach who started his initial work on LSD training back in the 1920s. The intensity for LSD training will typically vary between 60% and 80% of the maximal heart rate. Distance, not speed, becomes the major objective. Highly conditioned competitive distance runners who use LSD techniques will run 10 to 30 miles per day, or between 100 and 200 miles per week. Elite runners capable of sustaining a 5-minute-per-mile pace in marathons will train at a 6-to-7-minutes-per-mile pace. There is one major problem with this form of training. While the acute stress is low, due to the low intensity of the workout, the chronic stresses are considerable, and injuries are not at all uncommon. The possibility of injury is a serious consideration for those who are training over 10 miles per day. Those running under 5 miles per day are not nearly as vulnerable to the "overuse" types of injuries.

The low-intensity continuous training is ideal for the individual who is just starting an exercise program for its health-related benefits. The intensity of exercise is low and is of much less risk than either the high-intensity continuous or the interval training procedures. This is an important consideration since vigorous or burst-type activity in the older individual who has been sedentary is potentially dangerous. The low-intensity exercise is also more tolerable for those who are older or who have not been exercising on a regular basis. The higher-intensity exercises are very stressful and may discourage the individual who is attempting to regain regular exercise habits. Low-intensity exercise is typically only moderate to brisk walking for the average 50-year-old male who has been sedentary for over half of his life. It may take him 6 months to a year to advance from a walking to a jogging program using the low-intensity continuous training approach. However, the low intensity and gradual progression may be a major factor in whether that individual adheres to his program or becomes another fitness program dropout.

Another form of continuous training which is used almost exclusively in the training of athletes is Fartlek training, or speed play. Originally developed in Sweden, Fartlek training involves varying the pace from a very slow and leisurely jog to a high-speed, all-out run, but the speed changes come at the will of the athlete. This is a free form of training where distance and time have no relevance. The main goal is for the individual to have fun and enjoy himself. This type of training is usually performed in the country where there are a variety of hills. This form of training is most often used as relief from other more structured forms of training. While it is considered as a form of continuous training, the variations in pace are similar to interval training.

Circuit Training

In 1953, Professors R. E. Morgan and G. T. Adamson of the University of Leeds, in England, introduced a new training procedure which was quite popular during the late 1950s and the early 1960s, which is referred to as *circuit training*. This was an intriguing development, since it incorporated strength and muscular endurance, flexibility, and cardiorespiratory endurance activities into a single program of exercise. Also, it provided a degree of versatility which allowed the program to be varied to meet the specific needs of the individual, or of any one group, such as a group of athletes. With so many positive attributes, it is surprising that

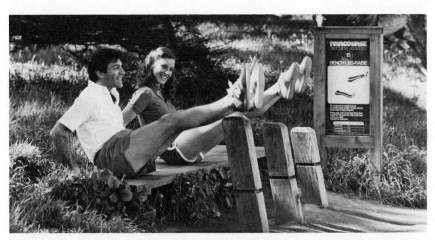

FIGURE 19. Parcourse station (Photo courtesy of Michael F. Calhoun, PARCOURSE LTD., P. O. Box 99589, San Francisco, California 94109)

this form of training hasn't become more popular. During the past few years, a form of circuit training adapted to the outdoors has been developed and is now being promoted widely throughout the United States. Parcourse is the trade name in the United States, but the concept or idea was originally developed in Switzerland. The Parcourse Fitness Circuit consists of a series of 18 exercise stations, situated varying distances from one another (See Figure 19). From the start of the course, the individual runs, jogs, or walks to the first station, where he performs a particular exercise—*e.g.*, touching the toes 6 consecutive times—and then moves as quickly as possible to the second station, where he performs the next exercise, *e.g.*, 25 sit-ups. This continues until the individual has been through all 18 stations. The course is designed to start out slow (warm-up) and gradually build to a fairly strenuous level of exercise (endurance conditioning). It concludes by gradually reducing the intensity of exercise back to low levels (cool-down).

Originally, circuit training was set up inside gymnasiums, exercise rooms, and hallways, or outside on courts, fields, and rooftops. There are usually 6 to 10 stations in a circuit, although this number will vary in direct proportion to the availability of space. The main goal is to complete the circuit as rapidly as possible, with improvement being demonstrated either by a decrease in the total time it takes to complete the circuit, or by increasing the amount of work accomplished at each station, or both. Since the goal is to complete the circuit as quickly as possible, the farther the distance between the stations, the greater the cardiorespiratory endurance conditioning benefits. An example of a circuit training circuit is provided in Table 9 (p. 118).

TABLE 9. Example of a circuit training circuit

STATION	EXERCISE	WEIGHT, LBS.	RED CIRCUIT REPETITIONS			WEIGHT, LBS.	BLUE CIRCUIT REPETITIONS		
			1	2	3		1	2	3
1	Toe Touches	—	8	10	12	—	15	17	19
2	Chins	—	1	3	5	—	7	9	10
3	Bench Press	60	8	10	12	80	8	10	12
4	Stair Climb	—	4	6	8	—	10	12	14
5	Curl	35	8	10	12	45	8	10	12
6	Half Squat	80	9	12	15	95	12	14	16
7	Sit-Up	—	10	14	18	—	20	25	30
8	Stair Climb	—	4	6	8	—	10	12	14

TARGET TIMES   RED-23 minutes   BLUE-25 minutes

Various levels are established, depending on the skill level and the ability of the group. In Table 9, the red and the blue circuits indicate two levels, with three steps at each level. The number of levels, steps per level, the range of difficulty for each exercise station, and the specific exercise for each station are determined on the basis of the needs of that group of individuals for which the circuit was being developed. There would obviously be a considerable difference between the needs of a group of high school football players and a group of middle-aged women just beginning a fitness program. In the example provided in Table 9, the person just beginning a circuit training program would start with Red-1. He would complete the circuit three times without stopping, attempting to finish in less than 23 minutes, the target time for the Red level. When he can complete three circuits in less than 23 minutes, he moves to the next step, Red-2. After months of training he will have worked his way up to the Blue level or higher.

Circuit training offers a unique training experience. First, it emphasizes more than one component of fitness, so it could be classified as a total fitness activity. Second, it provides an interesting training environment since there is the opportunity for daily competition against the established times in addition to seeing continuous progress. This would be a challenge and a strong motivation for most athletes. Lastly, the circuit training program can be modified to meet the needs of the individual or the group, and it can accommodate large groups of individuals at a relatively low expense.

While circuit training is traditionally conducted indoors within a relatively small area, the Vita Parcourse idea, which originated in Switzerland, takes the circuit training concept outside. In Switzerland and the Scandinavian countries, the total circuit may be 1 to 5 miles in length, with stations every 400 yards to 1 mile. These courses are typically located in beautiful parks or in the country where there are many trees and hills. The individual walks, jogs, or runs the distance between stations, stops at each station to perform the specified number of repetitions of a single exercise, which emphasizes either strength, flexibility or muscular endurance, and then moves on to the next station.

Combination Programs

Most training programs do not rely exclusively on any one method or system of training, but represent a combination or blend of two or more systems. Combination programs provide variety, and since boredom is a real hazard of any intense training program, this variety reduces the chances of boredom and enhances the chances that the individual will adhere to his training program. For the recreational athlete, who doesn't have the motivation of competition, variety is a very important factor. For the athlete, variety may, in fact, be essential for success. A survey conducted by *Runner's World* magazine, in which the top twenty to thirty runners in each event were polled, indicates that top-level or elite runners at all distances, from the sprint to the marathon, rely considerably on variation. The results of this survey are presented in Table 10 (page 120). In addition to clearly illustrating the variety in training patterns for any one race, this table also illustrates how uniquely differently the athletes train for sprint, middle distance, distance, and long distance events, both relative to types of running and training site.

Table 11 (page 121) provides an illustration of a combination interval training and low-intensity continuous training program which was designed specifically for individuals who are beginning a walk/jog/run fitness program for its health-related benefits. It starts at a very low level of activity, walking three-fourths of a mile in 22½ minutes, and gradually builds up to a level where the individual is able to run 5 miles in 35 minutes. Progression from one step to the next within any one level will vary considerably from individual to individual. Once the individual has properly identified the appropriate level and step for starting his program, he should be able to move from one step to the next every 2 to 4 weeks, providing he follows the program precisely, and works out 3 to 4 days per week.

Starting such a program involves considerable trial and error experience initially. First, the individual should define his THR or the THR range as described in Chapter 4. Then, he selects the level and step which he feels confident he can accomplish and maintain his THR or THR range. As he experiences his first workout, his heart rate response to this level and step will allow him to determine the accuracy of his choice. If he completed his first workout with little or no effort, and his heart rate response to the exercise was well below his THR, then he should move up one or two steps and re-evaluate the situation after his next workout at the

TABLE 10. Runner's World Survey* of the Training Patterns of Top-Level Runners

RACE	AVE. TIME	DAYS/WEEK	MILES/DAY	TYPES OF RUNNING** (% OF EACH)					TRAINING SITE (% OF EACH)		
				S.D.	F.D.	INT.	FLK.	RACE	TRACK	ROAD	C-COUNTRY
100 yards	9.8	5.8	4.8	17%	16%	49%	12%	6%	50%	30%	20%
220 yards	21.9	5.9	5.0	35%	12%	39%	10%	4%	37%	37%	26%
440 yards	48.8	5.9	7.5	40%	12%	35%	9%	4%	44%	33%	23%
880 yards	1:52	6.4	9.0	55%	17%	17%	7%	4%	28%	50%	22%
One mile	4:10	6.8	10.5	55%	19%	15%	6%	6%	22%	52%	26%
Two miles	9:00	6.8	11.0	58%	18%	11%	7%	6%	17%	60%	23%
3 miles	13:50	6.8	12.8	53%	26%	9%	8%	4%	18%	50%	32%
6 miles	29:00	6.9	13.0	59%	21%	10%	4%	6%	18%	63%	19%
9-15 miles	—	6.9	13.0	51%	21%	5%	15%	8%	17%	54%	29%
Marathon	2:26	6.9	13.1	51%	25%	5%	13%	6%	13%	63%	24%

* From The Complete Runner, edited by World Publications, Mountain View, Californ a, 1974, p. 306.

** S.D. = slow distance; F.D. = fast distance; INT. = intervals; FLK. = Fartlek.

TABLE 11. A progressive walk/jog/run program

LEVEL	STEP	WORKOUT DESCRIPTION	LAPS*	TOTAL TIME, MINUTES	TOTAL DISTANCE, MILES
		WALKING			
I	A	Walk ¾ miles in 22 minutes, 30 seconds	3	22½	¾
	B	Walk 1 mile in 30 minutes	4	30	1
	C	Walk 1¼ miles in 30 minutes	5	30	1¼
	D	Walk 1½ miles in 30 minutes	6	30	1½
	E	Walk 1¾ miles in 30 minutes	7	30	1¾
	F	Walk 2 miles in 30 minutes	8	30	2
		WALKING-JOGGING			
II	A	Walk 2¼ miles in 30 minutes	9	30	2¼
	B	Walk ¼ mile in 3 minutes, 45 seconds	1		
		Jog ¼ mile in 3 minutes	1		
		Alternate walk/jog for 5 sets	10	33¾	2½
	C	Walk ½ mile in 7 minutes, 30 seconds	2		
		Jog ½ mile in 6 minutes	2		
		Alternate walk/jog for 2 sets, then	8		
		Walk ½ mile in 7 minutes, 30 seconds	2	34½	2½
	D	Walk ¼ mile in 3 minutes, 45 seconds	1		
		Jog ¾ mile in 9 minutes	3		
		Walk ½ mile in 7 minutes, 30 seconds	2		
		Jog ¾ mile in 9 minutes	3		
		Walk ¼ mile in 3 minutes, 45 seconds	1	33	2½
	E	Jog 1 mile in 12 minutes	4		
		Walk ¼ mile in 3 minutes, 45 seconds	1		
		Repeat for 2 sets	10	31½	2½
	F	Walk ¼ mile in 3 minutes, 45 seconds	1		
		Jog 1 mile in 11 minutes	4		
		Repeat for 2 sets	10		
		Walk ¼ mile in 3 minutes, 45 seconds	1	33¼	2¾
		JOGGING			
III	A	Jog 1 mile in 11 minutes	4		
		Jog ½ mile in 6 minutes	2		
		Repeat for 2 sets	12	34	3
	B	Jog 3 miles in 33 minutes	12	33	3
	C	Jog 1 mile in 10 minutes	4		
		Jog 1 mile in 11 minutes	4		
		Jog 1 mile in 10 minutes	4	31	3
	D	Jog 3 miles in 30 minutes	12	30	3
	E	Jog 1 mile in 9 minutes, 15 seconds	4		
		Jog 1 mile in 10 minutes	4		
		Jog 1 mile in 9 minutes, 15 seconds	4	28½	3
	F	Jog 3 miles in 27 minutes, 45 seconds	12	27¾	3
		JOGGING—RUNNING			
IV	A	Jog 3¼ miles in 30 minutes	13	30	3¼
	B	Jog 3½ miles in 31 minutes, 30 seconds	14	31½	3½
	C	Jog 3½ miles in 29 minutes, 45 seconds	14	29¾	3½
	D	Jog-Run 3½ miles in 28 minutes	14	28	3½
	E	Jog-Run 3¾ miles in 30 minutes	15	30	3¾
	F	Jog-Run 4 miles in 32 minutes	16	32	4
		RUNNING			
V	A	Run 4 miles in 30 minutes	16	30	4
	B	Run 4¼ miles in 32 minutes	17	32	4¼
	C	Run 4½ miles in 33 minutes, 45 seconds	18	33¾	4½
	D	Run 4½ miles in 31 minutes, 30 seconds	18	31½	4½
	E	Run 4¾ miles in 33 minutes, 15 seconds	19	33¼	4¾
	F	Run 5 miles in 35 minutes	20	35	5

*Number of laps on a quarter-mile or 440-yard track

new intensity of exercise. Just the opposite approach would be used if the individual had selected an initial level and step which was above his capacity. Eventually, usually within several workout sessions, the individual arrives at his appropriate level and step. Progression from one step to the next within the same level, or from the highest step in one level to the lowest step in the next highest level, is also determined largely by the heart rate response to exercise. As the individual becomes better conditioned, his heart rate response to a specific level and step of work will decrease with each workout, although this may not be true on certain days because of complicating factors such as illness, lack of sleep, or increases in the temperature of the exercise environment. Once the heart rate response to a given level and step of work drops 10 beats or more below the THR, it is then time to move up to the next step. It is important, however, not to get overly concerned with time and distance, particularly if they detract from the enjoyment of the activity. For those who work best in a regimented and highly structured program, the program outlined in Table 11 will provide a gradual increase in fitness with many opportunities to monitor progress along the way. Lastly, it is not necessary to progress all the way through this program. Most experts would agree that the individual who is able to achieve Level IV, Step A, has a desirable level of cardiorespiratory endurance fitness. Any progress beyond this point would be solely for the enjoyment of the individual. Some may wish to progress beyond the highest level outlined in Table 11. For these individuals, additional training tips will be covered in Chapter 8.

ASSESSMENT OF CARDIORESPIRATORY ENDURANCE

As was discussed earlier, the best estimate of cardiorespiratory endurance capacity is the maximal oxygen uptake value. This is typically obtained during a test to exhaustion on a treadmill or a bicycle ergometer. For the individual 35 years of age and older, this test should be done only under the supervision of a physician. Few facilities are available where one could go to have his maximal oxygen uptake measured. Consequently, the only alternative for most people is an indirect estimate of maximal oxygen uptake. Over the past 10 years, research has indicated that the time to complete an endurance run of 1.5 miles or greater has a very close relationship to one's maximal oxygen uptake. Table 12 (page 123) provides the estimated maximal oxygen uptake for the specific time to complete 1.5 miles. The test can be run on either a track (6 laps), or on a 1.5 mile non-repeating course which assures that the total distance was completed, and was not a lap or two short. This test should be given only to those who are in good condition, or who have been conditioned to run that distance. The test is potentially dangerous for the sedentary individual who has been out of training for years. Pre-training is essential for

TABLE 12. Maximal oxygen uptake estimated from 1.5-mile run time*

1.5-MILE RUN TIME, MINUTES : SECONDS	ESTIMATED MAXIMAL OXYGEN UPTAKE ML/KG • MIN
7:30 and below	75
7:31– 8:00	72
8:01– 8:30	67
8:31– 9:00	62
9:01– 9:30	58
9:31–10:00	55
10:01–10:30	52
10:31–11:00	49
11:01–11:30	46
11:31–12:00	44
12:01–12:30	41
12:31–13:00	39
13:01–13:30	37
13:31–14:00	36
14:01–14:30	34
14:31–15:00	33
15:01–15:30	31
15:31–16:00	30
16:01–16:30	28
16:31–17:00	27
17:01–17:30	26
17:31–18:00	25

*Adapted from Cooper, K. H., "A Means of Assessing Maximal Oxygen Intake," *Journal of the American Medical Association,* 203:201–204, 1968.

valid results since proper pacing is important to obtaining good results. Those over 25 to 30 years of age should receive the appropriate medical clearance, as outlined in Chapter 3, prior to undertaking this test.

Other tests of submaximal intensity have been proposed as valid measures of cardiorespiratory fitness capacity, but each of these has major limitations. A number of step tests have been designed which estimate the fitness level of the individual on the basis of the heart rate response to a fixed rate of work. Unfortunately, these tests have not been found to be accurate in their predictions, although they are theoretically sound. For a given rate of work, the heart rate response of the highly conditioned individual should differ from that of the poorly conditioned, or even average conditioned individual, *i.e.,* it should reach a lower level during exercise, and it should recover at a much faster rate. Unfortunately, for some unexplainable reason, those step tests which are presently available do not accurately sense the differences in fitness between individuals. Submaximal tests have also been developed for the bicycle ergometer. The individual rides the stationary bicycle at two or three different work loads, and his steady–state heart rate for each work load is recorded and is then plotted on a graph relative to the work load from which that heart rate was obtained. The slope of the resulting curve provides an estimate of the relative fitness of the individual, with the steep slope representing low fitness, and the gradual slope representing high fitness. Again, the theoretical basis for such tests are sound, but the tests themselves do not provide very realistic estimates in actual practice. There is a real need to develop an inexpensive submaximal test of maximal oxygen uptake, or cardiorespiratory endurance capacity, which could be either self-administered, or administered by the nurse, physician, or the physical educator.

Once the maximal oxygen uptake has been estimated, Table 7 in Chapter 3 can be consulted to determine the significance of the resulting value. Generally, a value in excess of 50 ml/kg•min for men, and 45 ml/kg•min for women 20 to 39 years of age is considered to be very good, and possibly a desirable level to set as a goal if one's present fitness level falls below that level. For each decade above 39 years of age, the above target values should be reduced by 10%. As an example, a 55-year-old-woman would have a target value of 36 ml/kg•min (45 ml/kg•min − 20% of 45 ml/kg•min or 45 − 9 =36 ml/kg•min).

7

Training for Strength, Power, and Muscular Endurance

INTRODUCTION

For many years, strength was considered to be the cornerstone of physical fitness. Individuals who spent many hours per week lifting weights, increasing their strength, and developing large bulky muscles were considered to be the epitome of health and fitness. It is now known that the individual with the highly developed cardiovascular and respiratory systems represents the gold standard for health. This is somewhat ironic since the focus has shifted from the weightlifter to the distance runner, almost exact opposites in body physique. This change in focus in no way lessens the importance of strength as a primary component of physical fitness. Interestingly, it is no longer unusual for the distance runner to be seen in the gym or weight room working on the development of both upper body and lower body strength. Likewise, weightlifters and body builders are now starting to become interested in distance running!

Throughout the earlier chapters of this book, the terms strength, power, and muscular endurance have been used, but they haven't been clearly defined. These three terms are sometimes used interchangeably, but this is incorrect since each has a distinct meaning of its own. Muscular strength traditionally refers to the ability of the muscle or group of muscles to exert force. In most cases, the term "strength" is used in reference to one's ultimate ability or maximum strength. Thus, when one's strength is measured, the resulting value implies specifically that individual's maximum strength for a particular movement. One simple way of quantifying strength is to determine the maximum weight an individual can lift for a particular exercise, *e.g.,* bench press. Thus, to determine one's bench-press strength, that individual would select a weight he felt he could lift just once, and then be given the opportunity to attempt to lift that weight. If he was unsuccessful, weight would be taken off until that point is reached when he could lift the weight just a single time. If the individual was successful the first time, and, in fact, felt he could have lifted considerably more, then weight is added until he reaches that point where he can lift that weight only once. This is referred to as the one-repetition maximum, or 1-RM. Assuming two individuals were given this same bench-press strength test, and one had a maximum ability of 200 pounds, while the other attained only 100 pounds, then the first individual would be twice as strong as the second.

Power is simply the product of stength and speed. If both individuals in the preceding example had identical 1-RM bench-press values of 200 pounds, but the one individual was able to push his 200 pounds up to full extension in only half the time of the other individual, then he would have twice the power for that specific lift, if the distance the weight was lifted was the same, *e.g.,* 200 pounds per 1 second and 200 pounds per 2 seconds, over a distance of 2 feet, provides an estimated power output of 400 foot-pounds/second (200 × 2/1) and 200 foot-pounds/second (200 × 2/2), respectively. It is not at all unusual to watch two professional football players square off in friendly competition to determine who has the greatest bench-press strength. Once that contest has been decided, and a clear winner is established, these two individuals will go out to the practice football field, and the weaker man of the two is consistantly able to beat his stronger counterpart in line play. Football is a power game, and strength does the player little good unless it can be applied explosively over a very short period of time. Most sports are power sports, and while strength is the primary ingredient of power, the concept of speed must also receive attention. This will be a major point of discussion later in this chapter in the section on specificity of training.

Muscular endurance was defined in the previous chapter to distinguish it from cardiorespiratory endurance. The former is a local factor, while the latter refers to total body endurance. Using again the example of the bench press, where two individuals had identical 1-RM values of 200 pounds, when given 75% of their 1-RM, or 150 pounds, and asked to lift the 150-pound weight as many times as possible, the resulting number of complete repetitions would be a good index of muscular endurance. If one individual could complete 10 repetitions and the other only 5, then the former would have twice the muscular endurance for that specific lift. To summarize, the three terms can be illustrated with 3 subjects as follows:

Bench Press	Subject A	Subject B	Subject C
Strength	100 pounds	200 pounds	200 pounds
Power	100 pounds lifted 2 feet/0.5 second, or	200 pounds lifted 2 feet/2 seconds, or	200 pounds lifted 2 feet/second, or
	400 ft.-lbs./second	200 ft.-lbs./second	400 ft.-lbs./second
Muscular Endurance	10 reps. with 75 lbs.	10 reps. with 150 lbs.	5 reps. with 150 lbs.

While Subject A is the weakest of the three subjects, his power exceeds that of Subject B and is equal to that of Subject C, and his relative muscular endurance exceeds that of Subject C and is equal to that of Subject B. Absolute muscular endurance, which includes the weight lifted as well as the number of repetitions, would be much higher in Subject B, but would be identical in Subjects A and C.

MUSCLE TRAINING PROCEDURES

Before discussing the various procedures, systems, or specific pieces of equipment that are used to train muscle for improving strength, power, and muscular endurance, it is first necessary to define some additional terms. Essentially there are two major forms of muscle contraction: *static,* or *isometric* contraction; and *dynamic* contraction. Within each of these categories, there are *concentric* contractions, and *eccentric* contractions. Static muscle contraction, which is more popularly referred to as isometric contraction, is that form of contraction where there is no visible movement at the joint, even though the muscles are obviously in a state of contraction. As an example, if one were to walk over to a 500-pound barbell and attempt to lift it over his head, even though he knew his maximum strength for that lift was only 150 pounds, he would experience total failure. Obviously, the weight wouldn't budge. The individual may have applied the maximum force his muscles were capable of generating in that particular situation, and had the best of intentions, but no visible movement of the weight or of the joints occurred. This would be an isometric contraction. Dynamic muscle contraction is that type of contraction where the joint or joints and the resistance actually move. The lifting of the barbell in the above illustrations of bench-press strength, power and muscular endurance represent dynamic contraction.

Concentric contraction refers to the shortening contraction of the muscle, while eccentric contraction refers to the controlled lengthening of the muscle. This can be illustrated using the example of the biceps curl. The barbell is picked up and brought to rest against the thighs with the elbows locked out in full extension. The curl is executed by contracting the prime flexors of the elbow joint to raise the weight to chest level through complete flexion at the elbow joint. The biceps brachii was the major muscle involved and it performed a concentric (shortening) contraction to raise the barbell to the point of full flexion. The same muscle is responsible for lowering that weight through eccentric (lengthening) contraction. Had the biceps failed to control the return of that weight to the original starting position of full extension, the weight would have dropped rapidly as a result of the force of gravity, and probably crashed to the floor. In isometric contraction, again using the elbow flexion movement as an example, attempting to hold a heavy weight in the palm of the hand with the elbow flexed to an angle of 90° would illustrate an eccentric isometric contraction, providing the weight wasn't too heavy, since the effort was directed toward trying to match the downward pull or force of the weight. With the elbow in the same position, attempting to flex the elbow from the position of 90° flexion to full flexion with the resistance consisting of an immovable object such as a table which is bolted to the floor, would constitute a concentric isometric contraction, providing the table didn't move from its mountings.

When training the muscle, there are various systems or procedures which utilize either static or dynamic contractions. Each of these will be discussed in detail in the following section, but the definition of several new terms or concepts will be attempted at this time. Traditionally, strength training through the use of weights—e.g., barbells and dumbbells—has been referred to as isotonic strength training; the term isotonic denoting same (iso) tension (tonic). This term is, in reality, a misnomer, since the muscle is exerting different tensions throughout the total range of movement even though the resistance remains constant. However, the term is so firmly entrenched in both the popular as well as the research literature that it will continue to be perpetuated in this book simply for the lack of a better term which has universal acceptance.

Over the past 10 years a new system of dynamic strength training has been developed which uses the term *isokinetic* strength training. In isokinetic exercise, the term loosely denoting same (iso) speed (kinetic), the individual is contracting the muscle or muscle group against a potentially variable resistance. Again, using forearm flexion as an example, the muscles involved in this movement collectively produce a maximal force which is quite different at different points in the total range of motion of the elbow joint. The peak force development occurs at 90° of flexion. When the muscles contract as forcefully as they can at full extension or full flexion, the force generated is approximately only 45% of the maximal peak force generated at 90° of full flexion. Therefore, when lifting weights, the heaviest weight one can lift is limited by the weakest point in the full range of motion. Thus, a 1-RM biceps curl of 100 pounds would represent 100% of the capacity of that muscle at full extension, but would represent only 50% or less of the capacity of that muscle at 90°. In isokinetic exercise, the individual exerts force against a device which is set to move at a constant speed, and no matter how hard one pushes or pulls, or how much force is generated, the device will not move any faster than its pre-set speed. This allows the individual to exert maximal force throughout the full range of motion, providing he is motivated to provide maximal effort. Thus, the muscle can exert 100% of its maximum effort at each point in the full range of motion of that muscle, which is one of the basic points of difference between isotonic and isokinetic exercise. In isotonic exercise, the weight which is being lifted is constant, while the degree of effort provided by the muscles, or the relative effort, varies from maximum in the weakest portions of the range of motion, to moderate in the strongest portion of the range of motion. In isokinetic exercise, the muscle always has the potential for providing maximal contraction throughout the full range of motion, and as a result, the resistances will be variable depending on the force exerted by the muscle. This is one of several apparent advantages of isokinetic exercise. The second basic difference between isokinetic and isotonic exercise is the ability to control the speed of movement. In isotonic exercise, the speed is controlled by the relative amount of weight lifted, *i.e.*, the closer the weight lifted is to the 1-RM, the slower will be the speed of contraction. With isokinetic exercise, the speed of contraction is pre-set, and no matter how much force is exerted, the speed is maintained constant. This appears to be a major advantage of isokinetic training, but additional research must be conducted to confirm this as fact.

Figures 20 and 21 (pages 130-131) illustrate two devices which employ the isokinetic principle. The Mini-Gym device (Figure 20) utilizes a rope which, when pulled, is released at a pre-set speed. The speed of rope release is controlled internally and is not influenced by the level of force exerted during the exercise. This basic device can be mounted in any one of a number of different locations, allowing simulation of just about any exercise movement. Figure 21 illustrates a device similar to the Mini-Gym, which has been arranged for use on a swim bench. This device allows the swimmer to strength-train out of water, actually working on the patterns of movement used in the various strokes of swimming. This unit has a readout device which provides a direct digital display of the work accomplished with each stroke. In addition, it has a variable setting for controlling the speed of movement. Figure 22 (page 131) illustrates the Orthotron isokinetic training device. The Orthotron unit works on a totally different principle in providing isokinetic exercise. The speed control is accomplished by a hydraulic cylinder which can be altered to allow variation in the rate which hydraulic fluid flows through it; the speed of contraction increasing in direct proportion to the increase in flow of hydraulic fluid. Finally, the Cybex II isokinetic testing device, which was illustrated in Figure 16, can also be used for isokinetic training of specific muscle groups.

There are additional training systems which employ dynamic exercise, but which fall outside of the above definitions for both isotonic and isokinetic exercise. These have been classified or termed accommodating or variable resistance devices. Most of these devices vary the resistance by changing the mechanical advantage at various points in the range of motion. Nautilus strength training machines (Figure 23, page 132) use an extremely clever technique for altering the resistance throughout the range of motion. After studying the maximum force which can be gener-

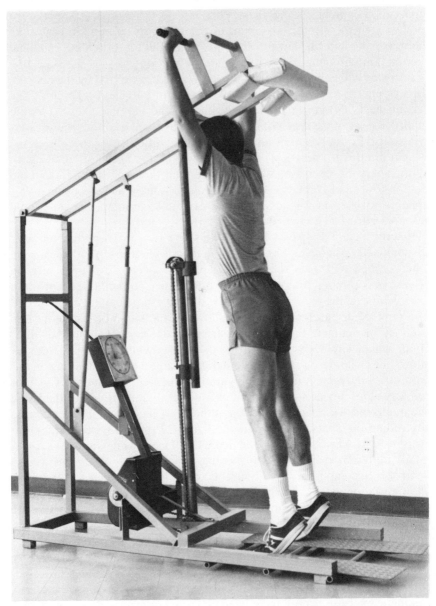

FIGURE 20. Mini-Gym isokinetic training device (Photo courtesy of Glen Hensen, Mini-Gym, Inc., P. O. Box 266, Independence, Missouri 64051)

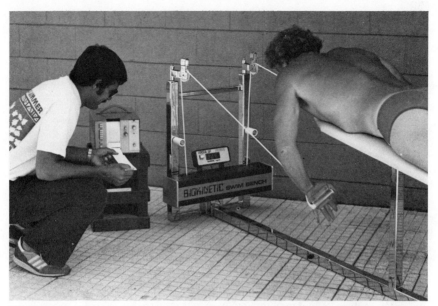

FIGURE 21. Biokinetic swim bench (Photo courtesy of Evan Flavell, Isokinetics, P. O. Box 6397, Albany, California 94706)

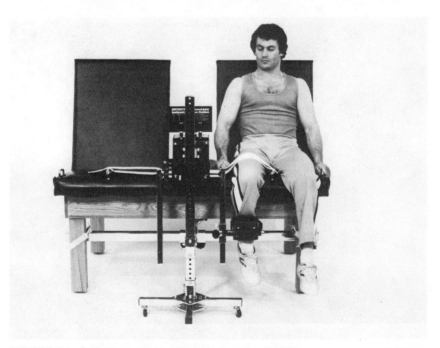

FIGURE 22. Orthotron isokinetic training device (Photo courtesy of David Hillery, Lumex, Inc., 100 Spence Street, Bay Shore, New York 11706)

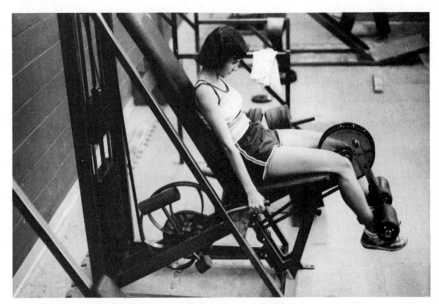

FIGURE 23. Nautilus variable resistance weight training machine

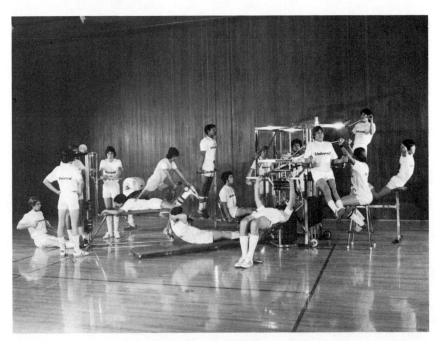

FIGURE 24. Universal Gym "Centurion," multiple station variable resistance training system (Photo courtesy of Norman Barnes, Universal Gym, Box 1270, Cedar Rapids, Iowa 52406)

ated at each point in the range of motion for a specific exercise, Nautilus designed a cam which attempts to duplicate the variations in force-producing capabilities of the muscle as it contracts through the range of motion. The cam can be seen in Figure 23. Universal Gym has developed a system for variable resistance training which is illustrated in Figure 24 (page 132).

Figure 25 (below) illustrates a totally novel and innovative approach to strength training. The CAM II system utilizes pneumatic resistance, which is achieved with compressed air and pneumatic cylinders. This unique approach to training provides a number of interesting possibilities for innovative training procedures.

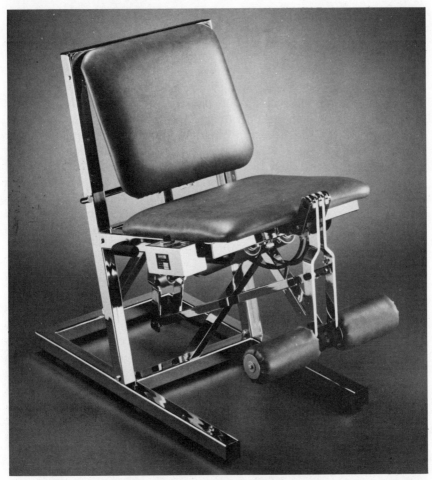

FIGURE 25. The CAM II pneumatic variable resistance leg extension device (Photo courtesy of Randy Keiser, Keiser Sports Health Equipment, 1627 E Street, Fresno, California 93706)

Finally, Dr. Gideon Ariel, popular exercise scientist in the area of biomechanics, has developed a computerized weight training system which is not on the market at this time. The concept sounds very promising, however, and could lead to major breakthroughs in the area of strength training.

With the above definitions, it will be much easier to discuss specific muscle training procedures. The following discussion will focus on static and dynamic procedures, with isotonic, isokinetic, and accommodating resistance exercises being included under the general category of dynamic procedures.

Static Exercise Procedures

Static training procedures were introduced in the early part of this century, but only gained popularity and support in the 1950s through the research work of two German sport scientists, Drs. Hettinger and Müller. The initial studies of Drs. Hettinger and Müller produced some rather remarkable results, indicating substantial gains in strength with only moderate training, with rates of strength increase which exceeded that of isotonic training. When these results first came to the attention of the American public, there was a widespread move to isometric training procedures. In their original work, claims were made that strength could be increased at a rate of 5% of the original strength value per week as a result of one 6-second contraction per day at only 67% of the individual's maximum contraction strength. When contraction strength was increased to 100% of the maximum contraction strength, or when contractions were repeated more than once, there was not a substantial increase in this rate of strength gain.

Subsequent research has been unable to confirm the magnitude of strength gains reported in this original research, but, nevertheless, substantial gains were still observed. These studies, and more recent studies by Müller and Rohnert, suggest that while one contraction at 67% of maximal strength held for 6 seconds does increase strength, greater improvement will result from 5 to 10 contractions held for 6 seconds each at 100% of maximal strength. It also appears that the muscle should be trained in at least 2 or 3 points in the range of motion, since several studies have indicated that strength gains are very specific to the joint angle at which training occurred. As an example, training at a 90° angle in the biceps curl leads to substantial increases in strength at that specific joint angle, but will result in only small increases at 45° and 135°.

Isometric exercises can be performed anywhere with little or no equipment, which is a very attractive feature of this form of strength training. In formal training situations, isometric power racks are very helpful. These racks can be constructed very inexpensively from 4-inch × 4-inch posts which are anchored upright either into the ground or on the floor. Matching holes in both posts are drilled every 6 inches, allowing a steel bar to be inserted through matching holes in each post. The bar can then be raised or lowered to the desired height for any one particular exercise. It is possible to perform almost all traditional strength training exercises with such a rack. The dynamic exercises which will be described and illustrated later in this chapter can easily be adapted to the isometric power rack. Isometric exercises can also be performed in the absence of any formal equipment. Pulling or pushing against immovable objects, and the use of towels, chairs or other similar objects, has provided the necessary resistance to movement necessary to train isometrically.

While the ease and simplicity of isometrics are appealing features, there are also problems which counterbalance some of the advantages. First, because of the simplicity, the individual receives absolutely no feedback relative to the magnitude of his improvement. When lifting weights, there is a continuous feedback as to improvement. Bench-pressing 120 pounds, 6 times on Monday and 130 pounds, 6 times on Friday of the same week, provides that individual with specific information on how much he has improved during that week. With isometric training, such feedback is not available. This presents two problems. First, it is impossible to determine how much force is being applied at any one time. While the individual may think he is performing at his maximum, there is no way of ascertaining this. Second, the lack of information with respect to improvement produces a serious problem of motivation. Without any concrete evidence that actual strength gains are occurring, there is the continuous possibility that the individual will abandon his program. Lastly, isometric exercise encourages the use of the Valsalva maneuver, where the glottis is closed and, with a full lung of air, a tremendous increase in intra-thoracic and intra-abdominal pressure is accomplished by contraction of the abdominal muscles and those thoracic muscles involved in forced expiration. The pressure builds to such a level that the major veins, returning blood to the heart from the lower body, either collapse, or their flow is greatly compromised. This reduces the volume of blood returning to the heart, and can result in serious cardiovascular complications. For middle-aged and older individuals, and for those with suspected or confirmed cardiovascular disease, isometric training should be avoided. The rhythmical contractions of dynamic exercise would be far more appropriate.

Dynamic Exercise Procedures

Dynamic strength training takes many forms, as was illustrated earlier in this section. In general, no matter which system of training, or which specific exercise device is used, there are several basic principles which have universal application. First, the principle of *overload* refers to the fact that in order to achieve a gain in strength, it will be necessary to stress the muscle or muscle group beyond that point to which it is normally stressed. As an illustration, a young boy is hired to load boxes from a railroad freight car onto a truck. The boxes weigh 50 pounds each, and for the first few days they present a real challenge to this young boy. After two weeks of working, he adapts to his job and the boxes no longer constitute a problem. He has adapted to this stress through a substantial gain in strength which was the result of his muscles being challenged by an overload. If the company for which this young boy works suddenly decides to shift to larger and heavier boxes, he will be in another situation where he is overloaded, and he will experience further gains in strength as he accommodates to this new level of work. The muscles must be loaded beyond those levels at which they normally work for significant increases in strength to occur.

The second principle of importance when training for gains in strength is the principle of *progressive resistance exercise*. This principle is best illustrated by a story from Greek mythology. According to legend, Milo of Crotona desired to be the strongest man in the world. In his youth, he began lifting a newborn bull once a day, and continued this daily ritual until the bull had achieved full size. Milo eventually became strong enough to lift the full-grown bull onto his shoulders and parade around the arena to the cheers of the crowds. As a muscle, or muscle group, becomes stronger, a proportionally greater resistance is required in order to continue to stress the muscle to the same degree to achieve further increases in strength. This is also illustrated by the example of the individual who just begins a weightlifting program. After the first few weeks he will have settled into a basic routine, and will have established the amount of weight he will use for each exercise, which will be appropriate for his level of strength. As he progresses with his program, he will have to increase the amount of weight he is using for each exercise. In the curl, as an example, he can lift 80 pounds only 6 repetitions initially, but following 2 weeks of training, he will be able to lift the same weight 13 or 14 repetitions. He then adds 5 pounds of weight to the barbell, and is able to lift the 85-pound weight only 6 repetitions. After an additional 2 weeks of training, the number of repetitions for the same weight will again increase to 13 or 14, which signals that it is time to add additional weight. Progressive resistance exercise simply refers to the systematic increase in resistance as the individual increases his strength. This principle applies to all forms of strength training and is closely related to the principle of overload.

In 1945, Thomas DeLorme published a paper in a medical journal which was to form the basic foundation for the development of systematic dynamic training procedures. While his initial interests were in physical medicine and rehabilitation, his system of exercise became widely accepted among athletes and others interested in strength training. DeLorme, and later DeLorme and Watkins, proposed a system which emphasized the use of heavy resistance and low repetition, with the intent of increasing strength, power, and the volume of muscle. The initial recommendation was for the individual to perform 70 to 100 repetitions over 7 to 10 sets of 10 repetitions per set. This was later revised to three sets of 10 repetitions each. With this system, it is first necessary to determine the 10 repetition maximum (10-RM), *i.e.,* the greatest amount of weight the individual can lift for 10 but no more than 10 consecutive repetitions. The first set is then performed at a resistance of 50% of the 10-RM; the second set at 75% of the 10-RM; and the last set at 100% of the 10-RM. As strength increases, the number of repetitions that can be performed is increased, and when they reach 15 repetitions or more, a new 10-RM is established and the weights used for each set are adjusted accordingly. As an example, if in the bench press, the 10-RM was 100 pounds, then the first set would be performed at 50 pounds, the second set at 75 pounds, and the third set at 100 pounds. If, after 2 weeks, the 10-RM increased to 120 pounds, then the weights for each set would be readjusted to 60 pounds for the first set, 90 pounds for the second, and 120 pounds for the third. Weights are usually adjusted every 1 to 3 weeks, depending on the initial level of strength of the individual, how intense he trains, and his overall potential for further gains in strength. The degree of improvement from one week to the next will vary considerably not only between individuals but also between any two exercises in the same individual.

While the DeLorme technique is still considered to be the basic technique in dynamic strength training, there have been many modifications. The Oxford technique was proposed in 1951 as an alternative to the DeLorme technique. In the Oxford technique, the individual performs 100 repetitions in 10 sets of 10 repetitions each. The first set is performed at 100% of the 10-RM, and each subsequent set is performed at a proportionally lower percentage of the 10-RM, allowing for the development of muscle fatigue. The technique has also been modified to a fewer number of total repetitions, usually distributed over 3 to 4 sets. In each set, the individual performs the maximum number of repetitions he can, so fatigue is progressive and accumulative.

The current state of knowledge relative to the optimal technique, or the optimal protocol within a particular technique, was recently summarized by Professor Emeritus H. Harrison Clarke, of the University of Oregon, in his comprehensive review of the existing literature for the President's Council on Physical Fitness and Sports' *Physical Fitness Research Digest.* Much of the work summarized in this particular issue of the *Digest* was conducted by Professor Richard Berger, of Temple University in Philadelphia. From the review, and subsequent research which has been published more recently, it would appear that dynamic exercise should be performed at 5-RM to 7-RM, for 3 sets each training session, 3 to 5 training sessions per week. This will optimize gains in strength and power. To optimize gains in muscular endurance, it will be necessary to increase the number of repetitions per set to 10 or more, and the amount of weight lifted would have to be adjusted accordingly.

As was described in the previous section, dynamic exercise encompasses a rather broad spectrum of training procedures, systems, and devices, from free weights (isotonic), to hydraulic cylinders (isokinetic), to air-resisted movements (variable resistance). The natural question to ask is: Which system and/or device will provide the greatest benefits? At the present time, each system has its own group of loyal adherents which makes many claims for the superiority of one system over another. Are these claims justified? From the limited research which has been conducted to date, no single system of exercise or specific piece of strength training equipment has been proven to be any more effective than any other relative to the ability of the system or the equipment to effect changes in muscular strength. It is entirely possible that the few studies which have been conducted have not asked the appropriate questions, or may not have been optimally designed to answer the appropriate questions. However, until such time that independent research can demonstrate a clear distinction between the results of training on one specific system or piece of equipment compared to one or more of the other systems or pieces of equipment, it must be concluded that no one system or piece of equipment is distinctly superior.

With all systems of dynamic exercise providing essentially the same degree of improvement in strength, how, then, does static exercise compare to dynamic exercise? From the limited research that has been conducted, it can be concluded that both static and dynamic strength training produce substantial gains in muscular strength, with little or no difference between the two procedures. Static procedures can be used during a period of convalescence from injury, since they, by definition, do not involve joint movement. This will greatly reduce the decrease in size and strength of a muscle or muscle group which typically accompanies inactivity. Due to the fact that static procedures will result in strength increases in only a limited portion of the range of motion, dynamic procedures will produce a more uniform gain in strength. Finally, dynamic procedures have been proven to be more effective in increasing both muscular endurance and muscular hypertrophy.

The following exercises have been selected to represent a balanced dynamic strength training program to be used with free weights. When other equipment is available, these same exercises can usually be modified to the specific piece of equipment, although the recommendations of the manufacturer of the specific equipment should be carefully followed. When strength training machines are available, they are suggested in preference over free weights for those just beginning strength training, strictly on the basis of safety. Free weights can be very dangerous if the proper precautions are not taken. When using free weights, there should always be at least one spotter, and preferably two, available to hand the weight to the individual once he assumes the correct starting position, to control the weight during the lift, and to take the weight from the individual at the end of the lift. Without spotters, even the experienced lifter can get into trouble as he gets tired and loses control of the weight. Most machines either have the weights controlled in a weight stack, or have been able to eliminate weights altogether. The muscles referred to in the description of each exercise are described and illustrated in the appendix.

Barbell and Machine Exercises

1. Standing military press

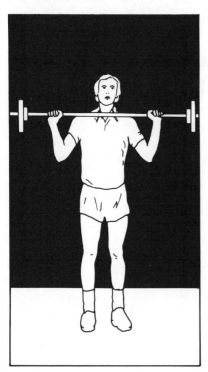 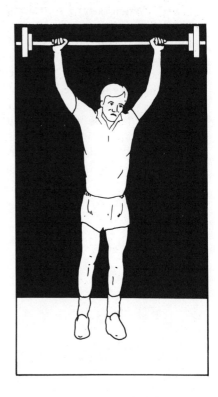

Purpose:	to strengthen the muscles of the shoulder and upper arm, *i.e.,* deltoids, pectoralis major, latissimus dorsi, and triceps
Start:	stand upright with the feet shoulder-width apart, the weight evenly distributed between both arms and held at chest level with the elbows directly under the bar, using an overhand grip, hands spread shoulder-width apart
Movement:	with the back straight, press the weight straight up over the head locking the elbows out at full extension, and return the bar to chest level
Note:	isolate the lift to the upper body, keeping the knees locked out in extension and the trunk and back perfectly straight. Specifically, *do not arch the back.*

2. Behind the neck press

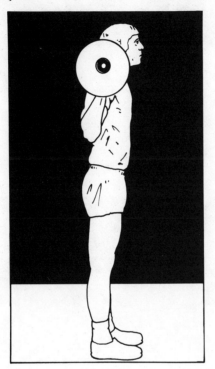

Purpose:	to strengthen the muscles of the shoulder, *i.e.,* deltoids, triceps, and upper trapezius
Start:	identical to the Standing Military Press
Movement:	with the back straight, press the weight up over the head to full extension at the elbows, and return to a position behind the head, touching the base of the neck prior to lifting the weight for the subsequent repetition; following the last repetition, return the weight to the original starting position
Note:	adhere to the same precautions noted for the Standing Military press

3. Bench press or inclined press

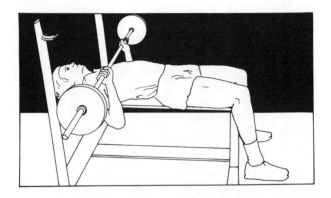

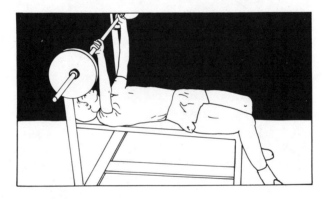

Purpose: to strengthen the muscles of the chest and upper arm, *i.e.,* deltoids, pectoralis major, and latissimus dorsi

Start: lie on a narrow bench with the feet spread apart on the floor, the weight held over head with the elbows locked in full extension, using an overhand grip, hands spread shoulder-width apart

Movement: carefully lower the weight to the chest, making brief and light contact with the chest, then push upward returning the weight to its original starting position

Note: isolate the movement to the muscles of the shoulders and arms, taking particular caution not to arch the back; the inclined press is performed in the same manner, except the bench is inclined to a 45-to-60-degree angle

4. Upright rowing

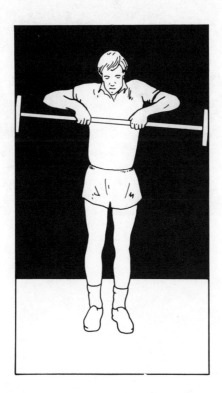

Purpose: to strengthen the muscles of the shoulder and arm, *i.e.,* trapezius, deltoids, biceps, brachioradialis, and brachialis

Start: stand upright, feet spread shoulder-width apart, and grab the bar with an overhand grip, hands spread approximately 6 to 8 inches apart, bar resting at waist level

Movement: lift the bar to the height of the chin with the elbows extended outward and return to the starting position

Note: isolate the muscles of the shoulder and upper arm; do *not* involve the back

5. Bent rowing

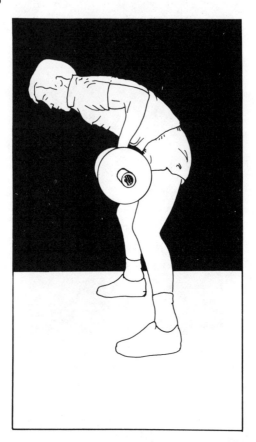

Purpose:	to strengthen the muscles of the shoulder girdle, *i.e.,* trapezius, latissimus dorsi, rhomboids, and deltoids
Start:	bend forward at the waist, back parallel to the ground, knees bent forward to approximately a 45° angle, and grab the bar with an overhand grip, hands spread shoulder-width apart, allowing the bar to hang down; place the forehead on something stationary—*e.g.,* wall—to help remove the involvement of the back
Movement:	with the bar hanging at full extension of the elbows, lift the bar upward until it makes brief and light contact with the chest, and return to the starting position
Note:	do *not* involve the back

6. Two-arm curl

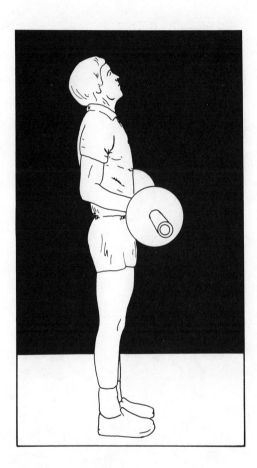

Purpose:	to strengthen the muscles of the arm, *i.e.,* biceps and brachioradialis
Start:	stand upright with the feet spread shoulder-width apart, the weight held at the waist or upper thigh level with an underhand grip, hands spread shoulder-width apart
Movement:	lift the bar to a position of full flexion and return to a position of full extension
Note:	isolate the movement to the arms; *do not* allow the back to arch

7. Reverse curl

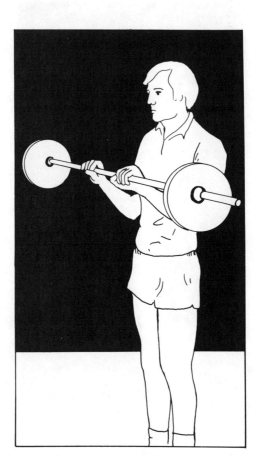

Purpose: to strengthen the muscles of the arm, *i.e.,* biceps, brachialis, and brachioradialis

Start: identical to the Two-Arm Curl, except use an over-hand grip

Movement: identical to the Two-Arm curl

Note: identical to the Two-Arm Curl

8. Lat machine pull-down

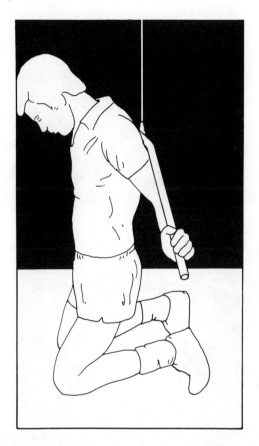

Purpose: to strengthen the muscles of the shoulder girdle and back, *i.e.,* latissimus dorsi, trapezius, and pectoralis major

Start: sit on a bench or kneel on the knees, keeping the back and head upright, grab the bar with an overhand grip, hands spread shoulder-width or farther apart

Movement: pull the bar down to a position where it just touches briefly the base of the neck and then allow the bar to return slowly to its original overhead position

Note: it may be necessary to anchor the feet or legs in some manner if the individual is particularly strong, to keep the weight from pulling the individual up

9. Lat machine triceps extension

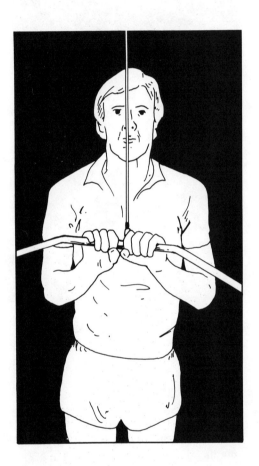

Purpose: to strengthen the muscles of the arms, *i.e.*, deltoids and triceps

Start: stand upright with the feet spread shoulder-width apart, grab the bar at chest level with an overhand grip, hands close together

Movement: press the bar downward to a position of full elbow extension and allow the bar to return slowly to its original position

10. Bent-arm pull-over

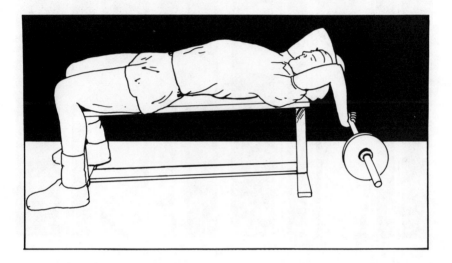

Purpose:	to increase the strength of the muscles of the chest, *i.e.*, deltoids, pectoralis major, latissimus dorsi, and serratus anterior
Start:	lie supine on a narrow bench, with the head at the very edge of the bench, grab the bar with an overhand grip, hands shoulder-width apart, with the arms fully extended overhead
Movement:	lower the bar slowly behind the head and downward as far as possible with the elbows coming to a position of full flexion; then return the bar to the original position with the elbows locked overhead in full extension
Note:	be extremely careful with this lift, as the weight moves directly over the face

11. Half-squat

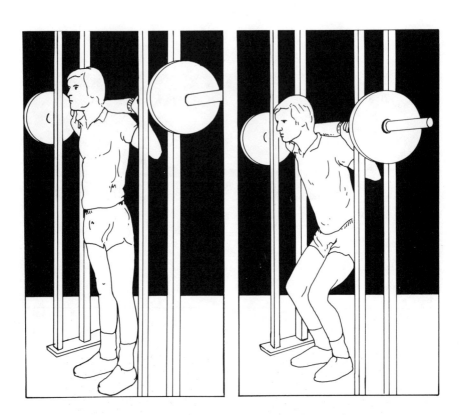

Purpose:	to strengthen the muscles of the lower back and legs, *i.e.,* gluteus maximus, quadriceps femoris, abdominals, and erector spinae
Start:	stand erect with the bar resting comfortably on the shoulders using an overhand grip, with the hands and feet spread shoulder-width apart
Movement:	lower the weight by bending at the knees to a 90° angle and return to the upright position
Note:	padding of the bar may be necessary to keep the bar from digging into the shoulders; do not exceed 90° of flexion! Have full control of the weight.

12. Hack squat

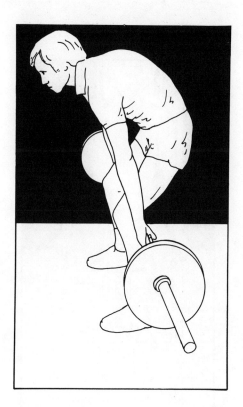

Purpose: same as the Half-Squat
Start: same as the Half-Squat, except the weight is held
    behind the legs
Movement: same as the Half-Squat

13. Leg extension

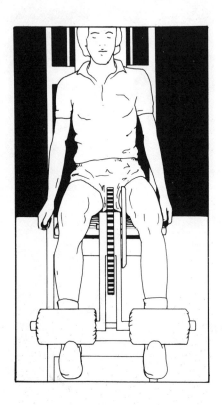

Purpose: to strengthen the muscles of the upper leg, *i.e.,* quadriceps femoris group

Start: sit on the edge of the leg extension machine with the knee flexed to 90°

Movement: extend the leg outward at the knee joint until it locks into full extension and then return to the starting position

14. Leg flexion

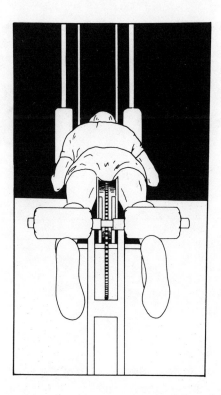

Purpose:	to strengthen the muscles of the upper leg, *i.e.,* hamstrings and gluteus maximus
Start:	lie on the leg flexion machine in the prone position with the knees fully extended backward
Movement:	flex the leg at the knee joint to a position of full flexion and then return to the starting position

Dumbbell and Free Weight Exercises

15. Weighted sit-up

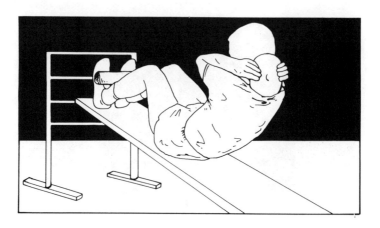

Purpose:	to strengthen the muscles of the trunk, *i.e.,* rectus abdominus and obliques
Start:	lie supine on an inclined board, knees locked forward in full extension, and a weight held behind the neck
Movement:	curl forward and upward slowly, touching the elbows to the knees, and then return to the starting position
Note:	this exercise may also be performed with the knees flexed to 90° on a slant board

16. Lateral arm raises

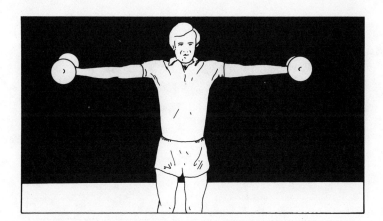

Purpose:	to strengthen the muscles of the shoulder, *i.e.,* deltoids, trapezius, and serratus anterior
Start:	stand upright, feet shoulder-width apart, dumbbells hanging downward along the side of the body
Movement:	raise both arms out to the side of the body to an overhead position, maintaining the elbows locked in full extension, and return to the starting position

17. Bench-lying lateral arm raises

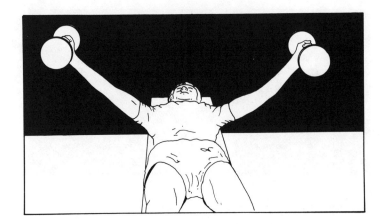

Purpose: to strengthen the shoulders and chest, *i.e.,* deltoids, pectoralis major, and serratus anterior

Start: lie supine on a bench with the arms extended outward to the side, and the dumbbells grasped firmly in each hand

Movement: raise the arms sideward to the overhead position, keeping the elbows locked in full extension, and return to the starting position

18. Neck flexion

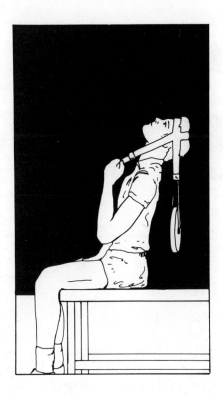

Purpose:	to strengthen the muscles of the neck and shoulders
Start:	sit in a chair with the neck in a hyperextended position and the weight attached to a head harness at the rear of the head
Movement:	slowly curl the head forward to the upright position and return to the position of hyperextension
Note:	control all movement very carefully by making all movements slow and deliberate

19. Neck extension

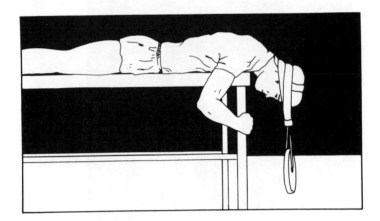

Purpose: to strengthen the muscles of the neck and shoulders

Start: lie on the edge of a table in the prone position with the head extended out over the edge of the table in a semi-flexed position with the weight attached to a head harness

Movement: slowly pull the head backward into a position of hyperextension and return to the starting position

Note: control all movement very carefully, by making all movements slow and deliberate

Muscle Soreness

There are essentially two types of muscle soreness. Immediately following a bout of intense muscular exercise, there is a transient soreness which may last from a few minutes to a period of several hours. This immediate soreness is probably the result of the accumulation of the waste products of anaerobic metabolism, and tissue edema, or swelling of the local area, due to the high hydrostatic pressures which force fluid out of the blood and into the surrounding tissue. This is the "pumped-up" feeling that the athlete experiences shortly after an intense exercise bout. The pain and soreness in this immediate acute phase is minor and causes little discomfort. Of greater significance is the pain and soreness which is usually felt from 12 to 48 hours following an intense bout of exercise. This pain and soreness can be incapacitating.

The muscle soreness which is felt from 12 to 48 hours after the bout of exercise is still not yet well understood. Several theories have been advanced, but they don't appear to be able to account for all forms of this late appearing or latent muscle soreness. One theory states that soreness is the result of small tears in either or both the muscle and connective tissue. While actual structural damage is a possible outcome of certain types of exercise, it is difficult to accept that all exercises where latent muscle soreness has resulted could lead to this level of micro-trauma. A second theory, proposed by Professor Herbert deVries of the University of Southern California, has been referred to as the muscle spasm theory. According to this theory, exercise leads to localized muscle ischemia, or inadequate blood supply, which causes immediate pain. This pain generates reflexes for increased motor activity, creating increased local muscle tension, which leads to even greater degrees of ischemia. He has collected research data in support of this theory, including the finding that static stretching not only helps to prevent muscle soreness, but it also provides relief to soreness when it is present.

Two factors have direct relevance to the eventual discovery of the cause of muscle soreness. First, muscle soreness is usually only present in the initial stages of training, *i.e.,* the first week or two, after which it tends to disappear. This observation is valid only if the training stimulus remains constant, for whenever there is a big increase in the training stimulus, there is renewed soreness. Secondly, there appears to be no muscle soreness associated with exercises which employ purely concentric contraction. Certain isokinetic equipment employ only concentric contraction, and no matter how hard one trains, there is little or no resulting muscle soreness. In one study, two groups of young men isotonically strength-trained using only the bench-press exercise. One group trained in the conventional way and had the usual amount of muscle soreness during the first few weeks of the study. The second group performed only the concentric phase of the bench-press exercise, *i.e.*, lifting the weight up. Two spotters standing on either side of the weight took the weight at the end of the full extension and lowered it back to the individual's chest, thus removing the eccentric phase. This group had essentially no muscle soreness.

From the above, it must be concluded that the actual cause of muscle soreness is still unknown. The lack of soreness with a leveling off in training and with the removal of eccentric contraction should lead researchers to a better understanding of its cause or causes. It may well be that there are several different forms of muscle soreness, which have totally different causes. This would explain some of the inconsistencies that presently exist in the research literature.

Specificity of Training

For most sports or activities, the closer the training activity is in actual execution to the sport activity, the greater will be the resulting benefits. Swim training greatly benefits the swimmer, but has little or no positive value for the runner, skier, or cyclist. Likewise, practice shooting of free throws does little or nothing for one's tennis serve, or putting game in golf, but it has big payoffs for the basketball player. How does this theory of specificity relate to strength training, when improved performance, not solely strength development, is the main objective?

The research to date does not support conclusively the concept of specificity in strength training, although the trend is definitely in that direction. If specificity does exist in strength training, what are the implications for designing strength training programs for each sport, or event within a sport? First, the strength training activity should approximate as closely as possible the movement pattern of the sport or event. As an example, the swim bench illustrated in Figure 21 was designed to allow swimmers to strength-train using almost identical stroke patterns that would be used in the water. Secondly, the strength training activity should be performed at a speed which approximates the speed of movement performed in the sport or activity. Since it would be literally impossible to strength-train at the very high speeds of movement that comprise most sport activities, it is then desirable to train at as high a speed as possible. Many of the more recent pieces of equipment have an adjustment which allows variation in the speed of training. For those devices without speed controls, the resistance is simply reduced to allow for faster contractions. It is postulated that the high-speed training is essential for the development of power.

Since the theory of specificity is not fully confirmed in the area of strength training, it would appear wise to build a solid foundation of traditional strength first, and then venture into more specific training. A combination of general and specific training may well provide the best all-around benefits for athletic performance. The ultimate criteria of success from any strength training program which is being used to better prepare an athlete for his sport is the improvement in his performance in that sport. To gain strength without an improvement in performance would indicate that the strength training program was an inefficient use of time.

ASSESSMENT OF STRENGTH, POWER, AND MUSCULAR ENDURANCE

In the research laboratory, a number of instruments have been devised to assess strength, power, and muscular endurance. The Cybex II isokinetic testing device, which is illustrated in Figure 16 (page 71), is presently the most sophisticated testing device available, providing a graphic recording of the individual's torque or strength at each point in the range of motion; a curve from which power can be measured; and a recording of sequential contractions showing the onset of fatigue, which is an index of muscular endurance. Tensiometers and dynamometers are also laboratory devices for assessing peak muscular strength.

One of the best tests of strength, however, is the one repetition maximum (1-RM), which was defined in the introduction to this chapter as the greatest amount of weight the individual can lift just once, for any one specific exercise. The procedure for measuring the 1-RM for any one lift or exercise was detailed earlier. Table 13 (below) provides what are considered to be 1-RM strength values for males and females on the basis of weight, for the bench press, standing press, curl, and leg press. Since strength decreases with age starting at about 40 years, these optimal values should be reduced by 10% for each decade beyond 30 to 39

TABLE 13. Optimal strength values for various body weights (based on the 1-RM test)

BODY WEIGHT lbs.	BENCH PRESS		STANDING PRESS		CURL		LEG PRESS	
	Male	Female	Male	Female	Male	Female	Male	Female
80	80	56	53	37	40	28	160	112
100	100	70	67	47	50	35	200	140
120	120	84	80	56	60	42	240	168
140	140	98	93	65	70	49	280	196
160	160	112	107	75	80	56	320	224
180	180	126	120	84	90	63	360	252
200	200	140	133	93	100	70	400	280
220	220	154	147	103	110	77	440	308
240	240	168	160	112	120	84	480	336

years—*i.e.*, 40 to 49 reduce values by 10%, 50 to 59 reduce by 20%, 60 to 69 reduce by 30%, and 70 to 79 reduce by 40%.

Power is very difficult, if not impossible, to measure outside the laboratory. Tests such as vertical jump, standing long jump, and softball throw for distance have been referred to as power tests, but their validity as power tests has yet to be established. Consequently, a simple power test cannot be suggested at this time. Current research will provide a simple power test in the near future. Muscular endurance can be measured by a number of field tests, including the maximum number of push-ups, pull-ups, and sit-ups. Another technique for measuring muscular endurance, which on the surface appears to be a purer measure of endurance, is to determine how many complete repetitions one can perform prior to fatigue or exhaustion, using a fixed percentage of the individual's 1-RM for that particular lift. This concept was also discussed in the introduction to this chapter. While this is a valid concept, norms do not presently exist since this is a rather new idea. Limited data, however, would suggest that 20 to 25 repetitions would be acceptable when lifting 70% of the 1-RM for any one specific lift.

Sport and Recreational Activities

INTRODUCTION

One of the major problems in motivating the general population to exercise is that many individuals simply cannot generate sufficient enthusiasm for exercise when their exercise program consists solely of conditioning–type activities such as jogging/running, calisthenics, and strength-training exercises. Conditioning-type activities tend to be boring to many people, and, as a result, the rate of dropout from programs that predominantly emphasize such activities is extremely high. Alternative forms of exercise which provide identical or similar benefits need to be identified and promoted. Sport and recreational activities are natural substitutes for conditioning-type activities, since they are pursued with the attitude of having fun. For most people, jogging is work, and as such is boring, while three sets of tennis is play, and is highly enjoyable. For a few people, activities like jogging are considered fun and enjoyable, but these people are presently in the minority. Our society has been recently brainwashed into believing that the only exercises which will truly benefit them are the conditioning-type exercises. Even more specifically, the misconception that any exercise or activity short of jogging is of little or no value has been widely promoted. Those in the majority, who do not like conditioning-type activities, hearing such claims, simply elect to remain sedentary. This is highly unfortunate, for there is a great deal to be gained from sport and recreational activities when pursued vigorously and regularly.

To briefly review a concept discussed in Chapter 4, there are two approaches in the use of sport and recreational activities. First, the sport or recreational activity can be used as the conditioning activity. Second, the sport or recreational activity can be used to maintain a basic level of conditioning once it has been achieved through conditioning activities. More succinctly, one can either play the sport or recreational activity to get into shape, or get into shape to play the sport or recreational activity. Even though motivation in the early stages of the program may be a significant problem, most experts now agree that it is a far better practice to spend several weeks to several months in basic conditioning activities to establish a desired level of fitness prior to undertaking a specific sport or recreational activity. Skiing, which is one of America's favorite winter sports, is an excellent example. Most skiers, even at the novice level, would not even think about getting out on the slopes without several weeks of pre-conditioning exercises, consisting of exercises to improve flexibility, strength, muscular endurance, and cardiorespiratory endurance. The same should be true for all sport and recreational activities. Attaining a reasonable level of fitness through conditioning-type activities should result in fewer injuries, increased ability to learn the fine points of the sport, game, or activity (basic coordination), and should allow the individual to obtain a greater degree of enjoyment from the activity. Using the sport or recreational activity to get into shape often leads to serious injuries, and can lead to serious, even fatal, medical complications, primarily of cardiovascular origin. A fatal heart attack on the tennis court, or in the racketball court, might have been prevented had the person achieved a reasonable level of fitness prior to seriously pursuing the sport.

RATING SPORTS AND RECREATIONAL ACTIVITIES

In the fall of 1972, the Opinion Research Corporation of Princeton, New Jersey, conducted a personal interview research survey of the exercising habits of the American population, sponsored by the President's Council on Physical Fitness and Sports. This survey included 1,939 men and 1,936 women, 22 years of age or over. On the basis of this survey, some rather striking findings surfaced. First, of the 109,000,000 adults in the United States at that time, 49,000,000, or 45% stated that they did not engage in physical activity for the purpose of exercise. These sedentary individuals tended to be older, less well educated, and less affluent than those who did exercise. When asked if they participated in any of a list of conditioning-type activities, the response, by age, is presented in Table 14 (page 165). These figures are misleading, however, for they do not provide the important information as to how frequently these activities were engaged in, how much time was invested per exercise session, and the intensity at which the exercise was pursued. As an example of the problems associated with such data, of those who said they walked for exercise, which was the most popular form of exercise, over half walked at least one to two times per week, but a substantial number walked less than once per week. For

TABLE 14. Adult participation in conditioning-type activities for age groups by percentage*

EXERCISE	AGE GROUPS, YEARS				
	22–29	30–39	40–49	50–59	60 and above
	Men				
Walking	36	27	39	39	46
Bicycling	28	17	18	13	4
Swimming	25	23	15	14	4
Calisthenics	23	13	10	10	5
Jogging	19	8	8	6	2
Weight Training	16	6	3	2	1
	Women				
Walking	51	45	41	38	33
Bicycling	28	31	20	10	2
Calisthenics	22	17	16	9	6
Swimming	17	16	13	5	4
Jogging	7	5	2	2	0
Weight Training	1	1	0	1	0

*1972–1973 survey conducted by the Opinion Research Corporation for the President's Council on Physical Fitness and Sports

those individuals that participated in sport or recreational activities, bowling was the most popular sport represented by 20% of the total American population, with nearly half of these involved in organized league or tournament play. Swimming ranked second, with 18% of the population as participants, although approximately one-half of these individuals swam less than one day per week. Of the remaining popular sports or recreational activities, golf involved 9% of the population; softball, 8.5%; tennis, 6%; volleyball, 5%; water skiing, 3%; and skiing, 2%.

The above survey represents the actual activity habits of the American population. How do these habits compare with a recent opinion survey conducted by the President's Council on Physical Fitness and Sports of seven highly qualified medical experts in the field of physical fitness? The results of this survey are presented in Table 15 (page 166). These seven medical experts were asked to rate 14 different forms of activity, which included sport and recreational activities as well as conditioning-type activities. The activities were evaluated with respect to their contribution to factors of physical fitness as well as to factors of general well-being, and a total score or rating was derived for each of the 14 activities. Comparing the two surveys, one looking at actual activity patterns and

TABLE 15. The ranking of 14 sports and exercises by seven medical experts*,**

	JOGGING	BICYCLING	SWIMMING	SKATING (ICE AND ROLLER)	HANDBALL SQUASH	NORDIC SKIING	ALPINE SKIING	BASKETBALL	TENNIS	CALISTHENICS	WALKING	GOLF	SOFTBALL	BOWLING
Physical Fitness														
Cardiorespiratory Endurance	21	19	21	18	19	19	16	19	16	10	13	8	6	5
Muscular Endurance	20	18	20	17	18	19	18	17	16	13	14	8	8	5
Strength	17	16	14	15	15	15	15	15	14	16	11	9	7	5
Flexibility	9	9	15	13	16	14	14	13	14	19	7	8	9	7
Balance	17	18	12	20	17	16	21	16	16	15	8	8	7	6
General Well-Being														
Weight Control	21	20	15	17	19	17	15	19	16	12	13	6	7	5
Muscle Definition	14	15	14	14	11	12	14	13	13	18	11	6	5	5
Digestion	13	12	13	11	13	12	9	10	12	11	11	7	8	7
Sleep	16	15	16	15	12	15	12	12	11	12	14	6	7	6
TOTAL	148	142	140	140	140	139	134	134	128	126	102	66	64	51

*From a survey conducted by the President's Council on Physical Fitness and Sports
**Each of the seven experts rated each activity for each component on a 0-to-3 scale, with 0 indicating no benefit and 3 indicating maximum benefit. A cumulative rating for any 1 component of 21 indicates maximum benefit is provided by that activity.

the other looking at the most desirable activity patterns, it is interesting to see that of the 55% of our adult American population who exercise, few of them are involved in those activities which will give them the greatest benefits. A 1979 Harris Poll conducted for the Perrier Company on the exercise habits of Americans indicated that only 15% of the adult population was engaged regularly in vigorous physical exercise, which was defined as expending 1,500 calories per week in sports and athletic activity, *e.g.*, jogging 15 miles per week.

It is apparent that the American population wants to be more active physically. Several recent national polls or surveys have confirmed the trend toward greater participation. There does appear to be a need, however, to direct this renewed interest in developing an active life-style into activities that will provide a higher yield. Obviously, it would be a mistake to force people out of an activity they enjoy and into another activity which will provide improved fitness and more health-related benefits if the latter activity is one which they will never enjoy. While the best health and fitness-promoting activities are the ones which should be recommended, moderate- or low-level activities are to be preferred to no activity at all. Providing the population with the basic facts as to the relative benefits of various sports and recreational activities will enable them to continue to select an activity or activities which they feel will provide them with the fun and enjoyment they are seeking from an exercise program, and to weigh that decision against the potential benefits to be gained from those activities.

SELECTING THE APPROPRIATE ACTIVITIES

There are many factors which must be considered when selecting a specific activity from the various sport and recreational activities. First, as has been repeatedly mentioned, the activity must be one which can be enjoyed and which holds the potential for maintaining the individual's interest and enthusiasm over a period of years. Second, the activity must be one which can be performed conveniently in the local neighborhood or within a short distance of one's job. Obviously, certain activities are not appropriate for certain regions, such as skin diving and water skiing for desert residents, or snow skiing for residents of tropical areas. Likewise, it is unwise to begin an activity where the closest facility is a 30-minute commute across town. Exercise facilities and equipment must be reasonably accessible, or the personal exercise program will not have a very good chance of survival. To be beneficial, the activity must be pursued at least twice a week, and even more frequently if possible. Driving long distances, having to wait in line to use a facility, and the unavailability of an appropriate shower and dressing facility are certainly undesirable and frequently lead people to abandon their exercise programs. Third, the expense of participating in an activity must be considered. Almost any activity will have some associated costs. These costs will vary considerably, from a $30 pair of running shoes for the jogger, to several hundred dollars or more for the downhill skier. It is advisable to seek out an experienced participant in an activity to determine what the average yearly cost will be. For some activities, the "hidden costs" are substantial, such as in boating. Fourth, select an activity that doesn't require assembling 18 or 22 bodies, such as baseball and football!

Since the focus of this book is on the promotion of improvement in health and fitness, the final, but most important, consideration should be the health and fitness benefit derived from participation in the activity. Professor Leroy "Bud" Getchell of Ball State University in Muncie, Indiana, has attempted to classify the various recreational and sport activities on the basis of their appropriateness for developing cardiorespiratory fitness, strength, muscular endurance, and flexibility. Table 16 (page 168) summarizes this general classification and expands on the information provided in Table 15. From both Tables 15 and 16, the relative merits of most popular sports and recreational activities are clearly presented. However, there are certainly exceptions to these

TABLE 16. The development of specific fitness components through various sports and recreational activities*

PHYSICAL FITNESS COMPONENTS				
Cardiorespiratory Fitness		Strength	Muscular Endurance	Flexibility
Continuous	Intermittent			
Bicycling	Badminton	Calisthenics	Calisthenics	Calisthenics
Canoeing	Dancing	Canoeing	Canoeing	Modern Dance
Cross-Country Skiing	Gymnastics	Cycling	Cycling	Fencing
Jogging/ Running	Handball	Modern Dance	Modern Dance	Gymnastics
Orienteering	Ice Skating	Fencing	Gymnastics	Handball
Skin/Scuba Diving	Jog-Walk-Jog	Gymnastics	Handball	Ice Skating
Swimming	Racketball/ Handball	Hiking	Hiking	Judo
	Surfing	Ice Skating	Ice Skating	Karate
	Tennis	Judo	Jogging/ Running	Skin Diving
		Karate	Judo	Skiing
		Skiing	Karate	Racketball/ Handball
		Racketball/ Handball	Orienteering	Strength Training
		Surfing	Skin/Scuba Diving	Surfing
		Strength Training	Skiing	Swimming
		Swimming	Strength Training	Tennis
		Water Skiing	Surfing	Water Skiing
			Swimming	
			Tennis	
			Water Skiing	

*Adapted from Getchell, Bud. *Physical Fitness: A Way of Life,* New York: John Wiley, 1979, 2nd edition

ratings. The level of playing ability will definitely influence the benefit to be gained from an activity, as will the intensity of effort. While handball may rate as a good all-around conditioning activity, if the person does not have the skill level necessary, or doesn't pursue the sport vigorously, few benefits will result. The information provided in these two tables assumes that the participants have the skill level and motivation to achieve the maximum benefits from that exercise, and in addition these tables are intended only as a guide. Table 17 (page 169) provides the relative metabolic costs of many activities.

TABLE 17. Selected activities and their respective MET values*

SELF-CARE ACTIVITIES	
Activity	*METS*
Rest, supine	1.0
Sitting	1.0
Standing, relaxed	1.0
Eating	1.0
Conversation	1.0
Dressing and undressing	2.0
Washing hands and face	2.0
Propulsion, wheelchair	2.0
Walking, 2.5 m.p.h.	3.0
Showering	3.5
Walking down stairs	4.5
Walking, 3.5 m.p.h.	5.5
Ambulation, braces and crutches	6.5

HOUSEWORK ACTIVITIES	
Activity	*METS*
Handsewing	1.0
Sweeping floor	1.5
Machine sewing	1.5
Polishing furniture	2.0
Peeling potatoes	2.5
Scrubbing, standing	2.5
Washing small clothes	2.5
Kneading dough	2.5
Scrubbing floors	3.0
Cleaning windows	3.0
Making beds	3.0
Ironing, standing	3.5
Mopping	3.5
Wringing wash by hand	3.5
Hanging wash	3.5
Beating carpets	4.0

OCCUPATIONAL ACTIVITIES	
Activity	*METS*
Sitting at desk	1.5
Writing	1.5
Riding in automobile	1.5
Watch repairing	1.5
Typing	2.0
Welding	2.5
Radio assembly	2.5
Playing musical instrument	2.5
Parts assembly	3.0

OCCUPATIONAL ACTIVITIES (cont.)	
Activity	*METS*
Bricklaying and plastering	3.5
Heavy assembly work	4.0
Wheeling wheelbarrow 115 lb., 2.5 m.p.h.	4.0
Carpentry	5.5
Mowing lawn by handmower	6.5
Chopping wood	6.5
Shoveling	7.0
Digging	7.5

PHYSICAL-CONDITIONING ACTIVITIES	
Activity	*METS*
Level walking, 2 m.p.h. (1 mi. in 30 min.)	2.5
Level cycling, 5.5 m.p.h. (1 mi. in 10 min. 54 sec.)	3.0
Level cycling, 6 m.p.h. (1 mi. in 10 min.)	3.5
Level walking, 2.5 m.p.h. (1 mi. in 24 min.)	3.5
Level walking, 3 m.p.h. (1 mi. in 20 min.)	4.5
Calisthenics	4.5
Level cycling, 9.7 m.p.h. (1 mi. in 6 min. 18 sec.)	5.0
Swimming, crawl, 1 ft./sec.	5.0
Level walking, 3.5 m.p.h. (1 mi. in 17 min.)	5.5
Level walking, 4.0 m.p.h. (1 mi. in 15 min.)	6.5
Level jogging, 5.0 m.p.h. (1 mi. in 12 min.)	7.5
Level cycling, 13 m.p.h. (1 mi. in 4 min. 37 sec.)	9.0
Level running, 7.5 m.p.h. (1 mi. in 8 min.)	9.0
Swimming, crawl, 2 ft./sec.	10.0
Level running, 8.5 m.p.h. (1 mi. in 7 min.)	12.0
Level running, 10.0 m.p.h. (1 mi. in 6 min.)	15.0
Swimming, crawl, 2.5 ft./sec.	15.0
Swimming, crawl, 3.0 ft./sec.	20.0

*Adapted from Wilmore, Jack H. *Athletic Training and Physical Fitness,* Boston: Allyn and Bacon, Inc., 1977

TABLE 17. **Selected activities and their respective MET values*** **(cont.)**

PHYSICAL-CONDITIONING ACTIVITIES (cont.)

Activity	METS
Level running, 12 m.p.h. (1 mi. in 5 min.)	20.0
Level running, 15 m.p.h. (¼ mi. in 1 min.)	30.0
Swimming, crawl, 3.5 ft./sec.	30.0

RECREATIONAL ACTIVITIES

Activity	METS
Painting, sitting	1.5
Playing piano	2.0
Driving car	2.0
Canoeing, 2.5 m.p.h.	2.5
Horseback riding, walk	2.5
Volleyball, 6-man recreational	3.0
Billiards	3.0
Bowling	3.5
Horseshoes	3.5

RECREATIONAL ACTIVITIES (cont.)

Activity	METS
Golf	4.0
Cricket	4.0
Archery	4.5
Ballroom dancing	4.5
Table tennis	4.5
Baseball	4.5
Tennis	6.0
Horseback riding, trot	6.5
Folk dancing	6.5
Skiing	8.0
Horseback riding, gallop	8.0
Squash rackets	8.5
Fencing	9.0
Basketball	9.0
Football	9.0
Gymnastics	10.0
Handball and paddleball	10.0

COMPETITION

It is fascinating to observe the phenomenal increase in young, middle-aged, and older adults who have turned to competition as an outgrowth or extension of their exercise program. Many individuals who took up racketball as a recreational sport are now entering tournaments both at their local club and at other clubs in the community, and enjoying the excitement of competition. Recreational joggers are turning to road races, and an increasing number are increasing their training mileage and intensity with the hope of one day conquering the full 26.2-mile marathon. The record number of participants competing in marathons in the late 1970s attests to this fact. While a field of 100 runners was considered a big marathon in the early 1970s, there were as many as 10,000 or more entering the major marathons in 1978–1979! Master's and Senior's competition has become extremely popular in swimming and track and field. These programs provide formal, high-level competitive experiences for men and women 30 years of age and over, with competition broken down into either 5- or 10-year increments. Official world records are kept, and there are yearly national and international meets in addition to numerous state and local meets.

Is such competition advisable? The answer to that question is a qualified yes. If the individual has been medically cleared for competition, and has been properly trained for his specific event, then competition can provide enjoyable experiences and will be a good motivator for maintaining high levels of fitness. One can't help but be caught up in the excitement and enthusiasm when watching these older athletes compete. The smiles on their faces, the appearance of their lean and healthy bodies, and the tremendous performances they are able to achieve are all indications of the positive nature of competition. However, some of these competitors fail to obtain proper medical clearance, and/or don't properly train for competition, and the result has been unfortunate for some, and even fatal for others. Several heart attacks have occurred either during or immediately following sprint-type activities in these competitions. Too often, the sprinter is the one who fails to properly train, for speed is such a natural or genetic factor. A sprinter can maintain a certain amount of his speed without maintaining his physical condition. An overweight, 3-pack-a-day smoker with high blood pressure is a likely candidate for serious cardiovascular complications from burst-type physical activity, even though he may still possess relatively good speed. Proper conditioning, preceded by an appropriate medical clearance, is essential for safe participation in competition.

How does one properly train for competition? For those in sports such as racketball, handball, and tennis, a good fitness foundation is essential, but once that has been established it is imperative that the focus be on skill improvement. To have an outstanding level of fitness without a high level of skill will win few, if any, matches! When the appropriate conditioning level has been achieved, the serious competitor in skill activities must begin working on the fine points of the game, including hours of practice to develop the appropriate techniques, coordination, and sense or feeling of where to be on the court or field. Strategy must also be a major consideration. In short, for those in skill activities, they must become students of their game. The higher up the competition ladder they climb, the more meaningful are the subtle, small points of the game. The reader is referred to any one of a number of excellent books which have been written specifically for the serious competitor in most of the currently popular sports for additional information relative to the fine points of a sport or activity.

For the serious runner, cyclist, or swimmer, skill is an important factor, but even more important is the level of training or conditioning. The competitive runner, cyclist, or swimmer must have a highly structured training program which will provide him with a means to accomplish a specific goal. The information in Tables 18 and 19 (page 172) was prepared for competitive runners. However, it can also be applied to competitive cyclists and competitive swimmers. In Table 18, the swimmer can approximate his training requirements by dividing the distance under the column "Event" by 4, using these new distances as his guide. The

TABLE 18. Training requirements for various running distances*

EVENT	TYPE OF TRAINING	
	Aerobic	Anaerobic/Speed
Ultramarathon	100	0
Marathon	90	10
15,000 meters (9.3 miles)	85	15
10,000 meters (6.2 miles)	80	20
5,000 meters (3.1 miles)	70	30
3,000 meters ($\approx$2 miles)	45	55
1,500 meters ($\approx$1 mile)	40	60
800 meters ($\approx$½ mile)	30	70
400 meters ($\approx$440 yards)	20	80
200 meters ($\approx$220 yards)	10	90
100 meters ($\approx$100 yards)	5	95

*The figures in this table represent the percentage of emphasis in training. These percentages will change depending on whether the athlete is in-season or out-of-season.

TABLE 19. Components of various systems of endurance and sprint training

TYPE OF TRAINING	AEROBIC	ANAEROBIC/SPEED
Interval Training		
Short Intervals (100–200 meters)	low	high
Medium Intervals (400–800 meters)	moderate	high
Long Intervals (greater than 800 meters)	high	moderate
Continuous Training		
High Intensity	high	moderate
Low Intensity (LSD)	high	low
Fartlek	high	moderate

cyclist should multiply these distances by a factor of 2 or 3. Again, as with the highly skilled athlete, the competitive runner, cyclist, and swimmer are referred to any one of a number of excellent books and magazines which provide much more detail on the design of training programs as well as racing strategies.

SECTION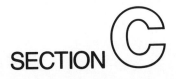

Special Considerations Related to Exercise and Sport

From the novice who has just made the commitment to start an exercise program to the elite athlete, there are many aspects of conditioning and competition which must be understood in order to have a safe, profitable, and enjoyable experience. The environment presents many unique challenges which must be faced intelligently, or the individual risks the possibility of serious injury. Heat, humidity, direct radiation from the sun, cold, and altitude are the major factors which will influence the individual as he exercises or competes. Understanding the problems associated with and learning effective methods for coping with these environmental stresses will be the focus of Chapter 9, which is the first chapter in this section. Differences in the responses to exercise and athletic competition between the sexes and with age will be discussed in Chapter 10. Chapter 11 will outline nutritional requirements for healthy living and discuss whether nutritional supplements actually facilitate or improve athletic performance. The final chapter, Chapter 12, will review the myriad of injuries which can result from sport and activity and discuss the various alternatives for effectively treating these injuries, in addition to ways of preventing injury.

Environmental Factors

It is a well-known fact that, in certain sports or events, the performance of the athlete will depend to a large extent on the environment in which he has to compete. The winning time in the Boston Marathon can vary by as much as 10 minutes or more, depending on whether the race is performed under conditions of 44°F and a light rain, or 92°F, high humidity, and no cloud cover, which are actual extremes which runners have faced in Boston during the past 5 years. A basketball team that trains and practices at sea level is suddenly transported to an altitude of 7,000 feet and finds that their typical fast-break offense and pressing-zone defense fall apart because the players are literally exhausted. Some sports or activities are not influenced to a great extent by the environment, since they are played or performed in a sheltered environment, altitude excluded. Wrestlers, gymnasts, and swimmers are seldom influenced by the environment since they are either performing indoors in a highly controlled environment, or outdoors in a pool which is also highly controlled with respect to temperature and humidity. A sport such as football can place extreme environmental stresses on its athletes, with pre-season practice beginning in July or August and competition ending in November, December, or January, depending on the level of competition, *i.e.*, high school, college, or professional. During the time span of the season, these athletes are exposed to the extremes of heat and humidity in most regions of the United States in the early part of the season, and the bitter cold, ice, and snow at season's end.

While the above examples are oriented toward the high-performance or elite athlete, the recreational athlete and the individual who is exercising for his health must contend with these same problems. This chapter will briefly outline the problems associated with exercising under various environmental conditions, and will then discuss how one can effectively contend with each of these stresses.

VARIATIONS IN TEMPERATURE AND HUMIDITY

The body is not a very efficient engine. For all of the fuel it uses, only a small percentage of this fuel is translated into useful work. The efficiency of performing various exercises or activities varies considerably, from less than 10% for swimming, to 20% or greater for walking, jogging, or bicycling. The energy which is required by the body to produce work is expended in the ratio of approximately 15% to 25% for the actual work produced, and 75% to 85% lost due to inefficiency in the form of heat, which amounts to approximately 80 kilocalories of excess heat at rest and up to 900 kilocalories or more during exhaustive exercise. This is illustrated by the increased warmth one feels when exercising on a cool day, or the extreme heat stress when exercising on a hot day. The amount of heat produced by the body during exercise is considerable. In cold weather, this increased body heat is welcomed. In warm environments, this increased body heat can be fatal.

As the body starts to exercise, the metabolic rate increases in direct proportion to the intensity of exercise, as does the additional heat which is generated from the body's inefficient utilization of its energy. Since body temperature must be very carefully controlled, there is a critical need to rid the body of this increasing internal heat load. The major adjustment made by the body to promote heat loss is the redirection or shunting of warm blood from the central core of the body to the periphery or skin, as evidenced by the red skin of an overheated athlete. When blood is brought to the body's surface, this allows heat to be lost more efficiently by *convection* and *radiation*. In convection, heat is lost or transferred from the body to a moving liquid or gas, such as cool air, while radiation involves the passing of heat from the body to the environment through electromagnetic waves. Body heat is also lost through *conduction,* or the passing of heat directly from the body to a cooler object, and *evaporation,* whereby the body sweats and the resulting water droplets are converted into water vapor. When sweat evaporates, there is a net loss of body heat which cools the surrounding skin. With the evaporation of every liter of water, there is a net loss of 580 kilocalories of heat.

Body Temperature Regulation

Body temperature is controlled by a small area in the very center of the brain referred to as the hypothalamus. The adjacent pre-optic area of the brain and special temperature sensors in the skin are also involved in temperature control. At rest, body temperature is regulated to a very constant value of 98.6°F, although the actual temperature at which this control is established will vary from one individual to the next. With exercise, the body readjusts its thermostat, allowing the temperature to increase to temperatures in excess of 100°F, and in prolonged exhaustive exercise to temperatures that can exceed 106°F. The resetting of the body's thermostat to allow higher body temperatures during exercise appears to be a desirable alteration, as the chemical reactions for energy production and the availability of oxygen are enhanced or facilitated at these higher temperatures.

Exercise in the Heat

When exercising in the heat, the effective heat stress is determined by the temperature, humidity, radiation from the sun, air movement, the intensity and duration of the exercise, and the extent of previous exposure to similar environmental conditions, *i.e.,* acclimatization. The fluid and mineral intake both before and during exercise is also an important factor.

When the temperature of the surrounding environment equals or exceeds the temperature of the skin—*i.e.,* 92°F to 93°F, convection, conduction, and radiation are no longer effective avenues of heat loss, and can actually become avenues of heat gain when the surrounding temperature exceeds the skin temperature. At this point, the body must rely totally on evaporation for heat loss. This works well for the individual exercising in hot, dry environments, but in hot, humid environments, the surrounding air is already highly saturated with water vapor, which limits the amount of sweat that can be evaporated. The higher the humidity, the lower will be the volume of available sweat which will be evaporated. In a hot, dry environment, the individual isn't even aware of the fact that he is sweating, because the sweat is evaporated just as soon as it reaches the skin. As the humidity increases, there is a decrease in the volume of sweat evaporated and the individual is suddenly aware of the fact that he is sweating. When the body's regulatory mechanisms fail or when the environmental stresses are such that the body can no longer effectively lose body heat, the individual is placed in a potentially lethal situation.

As the environmental temperature increases, there is a smaller gradient between the body and the surrounding air. This increases the reliance on evaporation, and, in fact, evaporation can become the only avenue of heat loss, as was described above, once the surrounding temperature exceeds the skin temperature. Evaporation requires sweating, so with an increased reliance on evaporation, there is an increased demand for sweating. Since the fluid lost through sweating comes primarily from the plasma volume of the blood, the total blood volume is reduced, imposing an even greater demand on the cardiovascular system. As the environmental temperature continues to rise, more blood is redirected to the periphery in an attempt to increase the cooling of the body's central core, while the rate of sweating continues to increase, further reducing the blood volume. With a reduced blood volume resulting from increased sweating, and a reduced central blood volume due to a redirection of the blood to the periphery, the total volume of blood available to serve the active muscles is greatly reduced, and the performance of the individual is greatly restricted. Most individuals are well aware of the fact that they just can't perform the same quality or quantity of work when they must exercise in the heat. In long-distance runners, the sweat loss may approach 6% to 10% of the runner's body weight. Man is capable of sweating up to 2 liters or more per hour. Up to an 18% reduction in plasma volume has been found in exercise with losses of 4% of the total body weight.

It is clear that environmental temperature alone is not an accurate index of the total physiological stress experienced by the individual during exercise. Humidity is an extremely important factor, for dry air is necessary for efficient evaporation to occur, and evaporation is the major avenue of heat loss. Air velocity is also an important factor, since the movement of air is necessary to continuously replenish the air surrounding the body. With a low air velocity, the air surrounding the body becomes saturated with water, and this restricts the efficient evaporation of sweat. The degree of cloud cover also influences the degree of physiological stress. Without cloud cover, direct radiation from the sun adds considerably to the total heat stress. Full or partial cloud cover provides tremendous relief when exercising in the heat.

One of the major problems associated with exercise in the heat is the resulting dehydration. As was stated above, up to 2 liters of sweat per hour or more can be lost during prolonged exhaustive exercise in the heat, which would be the equivalent of nearly 5 pounds per hour of weight loss. Marathon runners will typically lose 5 to 7 pounds during the course of the 26.2-mile race even though they drink freely during the race. Along with water, salts and other essential electrolytes are lost at a substantial rate. With the loss of every 1% of body weight, there is an estimated increase of 0.3°F to 0.5°F in body temperature. Obviously, everything possible should be done to decrease the rate of dehydration, since extreme dehydration has serious consequences which will be discussed later.

An essential part of any measure taken to prevent dehydration is to provide abundant fluids for the individual before, during, and following the activity. At one time, it was considered dangerous for athletes to consume fluids during practices or games. It was feared that fluid ingestion would cause severe cramping of the stomach and the intestine, so all fluids were generally withheld until after the practice or competition. It is now recognized that the practice of withholding water was the worst course of action that could be taken. Liberal ingestion of fluids during exercise is essential whenever dehydration is a potential problem. Fluid ingestion both before and during exercise has been shown to reduce the increase in rectal temperature as exercise is prolonged for up to 2 hours. For the same level of work and thermal stress, exercise with fluid ingestion results in a deep body temperature that is approximately 1.5°F lower when compared to the same situation with no fluid. One additional fact that has an important bearing on dehydration; man does not voluntarily drink enough fluid to replace that which he has lost. As a result, the individual should be encouraged to drink as much as possible both before and during the exercise period. Fluid breaks during exercise are to be strongly encouraged.

What type of fluid should be consumed before and during exercise? Water is readily available and cheap, but there have been major advertising campaigns and testimonials which encourage the consumption of specially formulated electrolyte solutions, and some are now promoting the use of beer as a fluid replacement drink. The most appropriate fluid replacement drink may, in fact, be water. Most of the presently available commercial drinks have too high a sugar content, and as the concentration of sugar in a drink is increased, its rate of emptying from the stomach is decreased. The most critical factor in fluid replacement is to get the water out of the stomach and into the blood. The water replacement function of a fluid replacement drink is much more essential than that of electrolyte replacement, or providing glucose or sugar to the body. Professor Carl Gisolfi of the University of Iowa has made several suggestions relative to fluid replacement which are soundly based on research. In addition to drinking liberal amounts of fluid prior to exercise, he recommends drinking approximately one-half of a pint of a glucose-electrolyte solution every 15 to 20 minutes during exercise. The glucose content of the solution should be less than 2.5 grams for every 100 milliliters of solution. The solution should be cool, slightly hypotonic, and palatable to the individual. Lastly, he suggests that a liberal salting of foods at mealtime will be sufficient to replace the salt which was lost through sweating during and following exercise.

One of the major problems associated with dehydration is the potential for heat disorders. When the body is unable to successfully adapt to thermal stress, there are three forms of failure which can result. *Heat cramps* is the least serious of the three, and is the direct result of the salt and water loss with dehydration. It is characterized by severe cramping of the skeletal muscles. *Heat exhaustion* is the next most serious heat disorder, and is characterized by body temperatures of from 101°F to 104°F, extreme tiredness, breathlessness, dizziness, and a rapid pulse. These symptoms are probably the result of a reduced sweat production, indicating the initial failure of the body's ability to effectively cope with the heat stress. *Heat stroke* is the most serious of the three forms of heat disorder, and is characterized by body temperatures of 105°F or higher, cessation of sweating, total confusion, and eventual unconsciousness. The victim of heat stroke will likely die if left untreated. When heat stroke occurs, extreme measures have to be taken to cool the body, such as immersion in cold water.

While the above discussion might lead one to totally abandon all unnecessary forms of activity when the environmental temperatures start to climb, it should be emphasized that exercise during the hot-weather months can be performed with minimal risk, providing certain precautionary measures are taken. First, exercise should not be performed during the hottest part of the day in the direct sun. Early morning and/or early or mid-evening are the most desirable times to exercise since the direct radiation from the sun can be avoided and it is typically cooler at those times. Second, the individual should wear the appropriate attire, which, in the heat, simply means to wear as little as one can legally get away with. For males, a light pair of shorts, brief socks, and shoes are ideal, and females can simply add a brief halter top. The more clothing that is in contact with the skin's surface, the more evaporation will be restricted, and the heat stress increased. Clothing should be loose-weaved and light in color to reflect heat. Under no conditions, even in the middle of winter, should one wear a rubberized suit. This has become a popular way to lose weight, but it is an extremely dangerous procedure, and the weight loss, while substantial, is all water loss, which is regained within the subsequent 24 hours. Within a short period of time, the air within the rubberized suit becomes fully saturated with water vapor. Since the temperature inside the suit exceeds the skin temperature, and usually exceeds the deep body temperature, with the air totally saturated, all avenues of heat loss are lost and the result is a steady increase in body temperature. The combination of profuse sweating and a rapidly increasing body temperature makes the individual who wears the rubberized suit particularly vulnerable to heat disorders. Third, the individual should drink liberally prior to starting to exercise, and he should plan to stop every 10 to 15 minutes for water, or some other acceptable fluid replacement solution. Fourth, the person should not exercise when the temperature exceeds 90°F to 95°F, and this recommendation should be reduced accordingly when the humidity exceeds 40% to 50%. The intensity and duration of exercise can also be reduced at temperatures below 90°F. Lastly, the individual should be aware of the symptoms of the three heat disorders, and should stop exercising when any symptoms start to appear. One symptom which was not mentioned earlier, but which is an extremely important one, is the sudden feeling of being chilled, including the appearance of "goose bumps," or piloerection. When this occurs, the sweating mechanism is starting to fail and the body temperature is being reset to a higher level, which could lead directly to heat stroke.

One additional precaution that can be taken to reduce the risk of exercising in hot weather is to become gradually adapted to the heat stress, a process which is referred to as acclimatization. Repeated exposure to the stress of heat results in a general adaptation which enables the body to better tolerate additional heat stress. While acclimatization will not enable the body to perform maximally under extremes in heat as it could under normal temperatures, it does enable the body to perform the same levels of work more efficiently in the heat, and allows the performance of even higher levels of work before the temperature regulating system fails. Total, or nearly total, acclimatization can occur within a 5-to-14-day period.

Exercise in the Cold

When compared to the potential problems of exercise in the heat, exercise in the cold presents relatively few problems. As with heat, cold stress is the result of factors other than just environmental temperature. The wind creates a chill factor, and the more moist the surrounding air, the greater the physiologic stress. A dry, still day at 10°F in the direct sun is much more tolerable than a moist, windy day at 40°F with complete cloud cover. *Runner's World* magazine published an article in 1973 which provided sound guidelines for exercising in the cold. These guidelines are summarized in Table 20 (page 182).

The clothing worn while exercising in the cold is very important. First, there is a tendency to overdress. It must be remembered that exercise will, by itself, create a considerable amount of heat. This can lead to profuse sweating if the person has overdressed. Sweat-soaked clothing in a cold, dry climate will lead to rapid evaporation with the resulting loss of body heat, which then can lead to severe chilling. Clothing should be put on in layers, and as the body starts to warm naturally as a result of the increased body heat accompanying exercise, the outer layers of clothing should be removed as necessary to keep the individual from overheating and sweating too much. Tightly woven garments will help to maintain a small pocket of warm moist air between the skin and the garment. Thermal underwear is recommended for the arms, legs, and torso in extreme cold, and gloves and a double pair of socks are also helpful. Since a great deal of body heat is lost through the head, a stocking cap or some other form of appropriate headwear would be most important. Males may wish to wear an additional pair of shorts or a pair of cotton briefs to protect their genitalia, since frostbite of the penis has been reported on a number of occasions, with the rather humorous documentation of one celebrated case in the prestigious *New England Journal of Medicine*.

TABLE 20. Wind chill factor chart*

	ACTUAL THERMOMETER READING (°F)											
ESTIMATED WIND SPEED (IN M.P.H.)	50	40	30	20	10	0	-10	-20	-30	-40	-50	-60
	EQUIVALENT TEMPERATURE (°F)											
calm	50	40	30	20	10	0	-10	-20	-30	-40	-50	-60
5	48	37	27	16	6	-5	-15	-26	-36	-47	-57	-68
10	40	28	16	4	-9	-24	-33	-46	-58	-70	-83	-95
15	36	22	9	-5	-18	-32	-45	-58	-72	-85	-99	-112
20	32	18	4	-10	-25	-39	-53	-67	-82	-96	-110	-124
25	30	16	0	-15	-29	-44	-59	-74	-88	-104	-118	-133
30	28	13	-2	-18	-33	-48	-63	-79	-94	-109	-125	-140
35	27	11	-4	-20	-35	-51	-67	-82	-98	-113	-129	-145
40	26	10	-6	-21	-37	-53	-69	-85	-100	-116	-132	-148
	Green					Yellow				Red		

(Wind speeds greater than 40 m.p.h. have little additional effect)

LITTLE DANGER (for properly clothed person); maximum danger of false sense of security

INCREASING DANGER Danger from freezing of exposed flesh

GREAT DANGER

Trenchfoot and immersion foot may occur at any point on this chart.

*Adapted from *Runner's World*, 8:28, 1973

ALTITUDE

The major problem when exercising at altitude is the reduction in the partial pressure of oxygen which is the result of the decreasing total pressure with increasing altitude. The low partial pressure of oxygen has relatively little influence on the loading of oxygen into the blood in the lungs, as the blood is almost completely saturated with oxygen until the altitude reaches between 7,000 and 8,000 feet. At 8,000 feet the arterial blood is 92% saturated with oxygen, compared to 97% saturation at sea level. This loss of only 5% in saturation will have some influence on the body's response to exercise, but the most important aspect of the reduced partial pressure of oxygen is the reduced gradient in partial pressure between the oxygen in the blood and the oxygen in the cells. The greater this gradient between the blood and the cell, the greater the driving pressure to literally push oxygen out of the blood and into the cell. As this gradient is reduced with altitude, due to the lower partial pressure of oxygen in the arterial blood, there will be reduction in the amount of oxygen that is transferred from the blood into the cell. Thus, increases in altitude are directly reflected in proportional decreases in the ability to deliver oxygen from the blood into the cell. This limits the availability of oxygen and reduces the maximal oxygen uptake and the physical working capacity of the individual in direct proportion to the increase in altitude. Activities of short duration are influenced little, if any, by altitude. In fact, certain activities, such as the long jump, may actually be enhanced by altitude, due to the thinner or less dense air providing less resistance while the body is in flight. Activities of a longer duration are definitely influenced by increases in altitude. It appears that the greater the aerobic component, the more the activity will be nega- tively influenced by altitude, and the higher the altitude, the greater the decrement in performance.

Can one adapt or acclimatize to altitude in the same way that one can acclimatize to heat? The body does acclimatize to a certain extent, but this acclimatization is never sufficient to allow athletic performance to duplicate that found at sea level. A major change that takes place during the initial few hours at altitude is an increase in the number of red blood cells, which is the body's way of adapting to the limitations in the delivery of oxygen to the cell. There is also a substantial loss in plasma volume which is the result of acute dehydration. Within a week to 10 days the plasma volume returns to near-normal levels. With the increase in red blood cells comes an increase in hemoglobin, and this facilitates oxygen delivery to the tissues. Maximal oxygen uptake is reduced substantially when first arriving at altitude, but it begins to increase with the increase in red blood cells and hemoglobin. This last response to altitude has led researchers, coaches, and athletes to postulate that high-altitude training might provide certain advantages to the athlete on return to sea level. Supposedly, every gold medal winner in the 1972 Munich Olympic Games running events from the 1,500 meters through the marathon were altitude trained. While a logical case can be made for altitude training physiologically, those few studies which have been conducted lend little or no support to this theory.

For the competitive athlete, recreational athlete, or the individual who is exercising for its health-related benefits, brief sojourns to altitudes above 5,000 feet will result in decreases in the ability to perform aerobic-type activities. Recognizing this, the individual should adjust his workout or pace in competition accordingly, with the understanding that both intensity and duration will by necessity be reduced.

10

Sex and Aging

INTRODUCTION

Over the years, it has become traditional to refer to females as the weaker sex. During the 1970s, in the United States, women became liberated, and new freedoms and opportunities were suddenly available. The 1970s observed the emergence of the female athlete. Where the athletic arena had traditionally been the domain of the male, females were now demanding equal opportunities, including budgets, coaching, facilities, equipment, and competitive opportunities. With the gain in popularity and total support of women's sports came a tremendous improvement in national and world records. Girls and women were beginning to close the gap between their records and those of the boys and men. On the basis of world records in the year 1978, the male was 9.3% faster in the 100-meter dash; jumped 16.9% higher in the high jump; ran 11.2% faster in the 1,500-meter run; and swam 7.3% faster in the 400-meter free-style swim. These are very impressive differences and tend to point to continued male superiority and dominance until a further check of the record books indicates that in 1976, East Germany's 15-year-old Petra Thümer swam the 400-meter free-style in what was then a women's world record time of 4:09.9, just slightly less than 3 seconds faster than Don Schollander's world record time of 4:12.2 in the 1964 Olympic Games. In analyzing the past records for the 400-meter free-style, Dr. Ernst Jokl has predicted that by sometime in the 1990s, the women will be swimming this distance as fast as men! Are women truly the weaker sex—i.e., biologically inferior—or do these differences in athletic performance reflect past social and cultural restrictions? This question, and other questions dealing with the female in exercise and sport, will be discussed in this chapter. In addition, the influence of age on exercise and sport performance will be discussed.

THE FEMALE IN EXERCISE AND SPORT

At full maturity, the female is 5 inches shorter than the average male, 30 to 40 pounds lighter in total weight, 40 to 50 pounds lighter in lean body weight, and is considerably fatter, 25% vs. 15% body fat. Up to the time of puberty, however, the average female is equal or greater in both height and weight, which is probably the result of the earlier maturation patterns of the female. At maturity, the male is characterized by broader shoulders, narrower hips, and a greater chest girth relative to his total size. These differences are due, at least in part, to the influence of the predominant sex hormones which begin to have their greatest impact at puberty. The predominantly male sex hormone, testosterone, promotes the growth of the lean tissue, having a major effect on increasing the muscle mass. Estrogen, the predominantly female sex hormone, promotes the deposition of fat. The mature female has higher amounts of essential, sex-specific fat in the breasts and other areas of the body. Thus, the female appears destined to have substantially more body fat and less muscle mass than her male counterpart, which would put her at a distinct disadvantage in the performance of most athletic events. Is this necessarily true, or are there other factors which haven't been considered?

Body Composition

The average female at full maturity (18 to 22 years of age) will have between 22% and 26% of her weight as body fat. The average male of similar age will have a body composition of only 12% to 16% body fat. However, when one looks at male and female athletes who have had similar training experience in competitive sport, the differences between the sexes is much less, particularly for those sports which have a significant aerobic or cardiorespiratory endurance component. Table 2 in the first chapter of this book provided information on the relative fat values of males and females in various sports. While the females have typically higher relative fat values for each sport, in certain sports there is an overlap in the range of values for the two sexes. In a study of 78 female distance runners, 12 had relative fat values under 10%, and nearly half were below 15%. Three of these female distance runners were at 6% body fat, a figure which is approximately the average for the world-class male distance runners. One of those three women had started a running program because of a weight problem! She eventually reduced her weight from 148 to 118 pounds, and, in the process, at one time held the best time in the world for the women's marathon. From this study, and others, it would appear that the average female is too fat, and that she has the potential to decrease her relative body fat values to 20% or less. The female athlete should attempt to drop her relative body fat to a level of 15% or less.

The higher values seen in the "average" female, and even in some female athletes, is more than likely the result of a sedentary life-style, which is acquired shortly after she reaches puberty. The male remains considerably more active than the female during the teens and early 20s, and begins to assume a more sedentary existence shortly after he marries, at approximately 25 years of age. Interestingly, the 35-year-old male has an average relative body fat of approximately 19% to 22%. Apparently, 10 years of sedentary living takes its toll in the male in much the same way it does in the female; the assumption of a sedentary life-style just comes some 10 to 15 years later in life.

Strength, Muscular Endurance, and Flexibility

There have been numerous studies which have confirmed the well-known fact that males are stronger than females. Recently, however, several studies have indicated that the earlier observations and opinions might not be totally correct. In a study of college men and women, men were found to be considerably stronger in both lower body as well as upper body strength. When strength was related to the size of the body, the strength of the legs was essentially identical in the two sexes. In other words, the quality of the muscle appears to be similar for men and women. Given the same amount of muscle mass, the expected strength would be essentially the same. With respect to upper body strength, the women were substantially weaker, even when strength was expressed relative to body size. For a man and a woman of the same body weight, the muscle mass of the legs is quite similar, while the muscle mass of the chest, shoulders, and arms is considerably greater in the man. Thus, strength is a function of the size of the muscle, or the amount of muscle mass, and is probably not related to the sex of the individual. Sex does contribute indirectly, however, in that the female will never have the absolute body size of the male, and the muscle mass in the upper body will probably always be proportionally less in the female. In studies where muscle biopsies were obtained from men and women athletes in the same sports, the relative fiber distribution was similar between the sexes, although the men appeared to have larger fiber areas.

Studies of women who have participated in strength training programs for periods of 2 to 6 months have demonstrated that women, like men, can substantially increase their basic levels of strength. In fact, women are likely to achieve greater relative gains in strength since they are typically starting at a much lower percentage of their ultimate capacity. Average increases in strength of as much as 30% have been noted following 10 weeks of weight training; however, some of the women in one particular study were able to double their strength in selected areas of the body. It appears that the female has the ability to substantially alter her basic levels of strength in a rather short period of time. In addition, studies have shown that changes in the size of the muscles with increases in strength are considerably less in females than in males, which is undoubtedly the result of differences in the concentrations of their predominant sex hormones. This is an important point, for strength training for women was strongly discouraged in the past for fear that those who did strength-train would develop large, bulky muscles.

There is very limited information available on the similarities or differences between males and females in muscular endurance and flexibility. Muscular endurance is typically highly related to the strength of the muscle or muscle group, and is therefore probably greater in males, although after a period of intense training there should be little, if any, difference. Traditional field tests of muscular endurance, such as maximum number of pull-ups, push-ups, or sit-ups, indicate much greater levels of muscular endurance in males. These tests, however, may not be an accurate reflection of muscular endurance as an isolated, pure component, *i.e.,* there may be factors other than muscular endurance which are causing the substantial difference between male and females. Flexibility appears to be much greater in the female at all ages. Even with considerable training, the female maintains an edge in flexibility. This is probably a genetically endowed advantage which could be the result of sex-specific hormone differences.

Cardiorespiratory Endurance Capacity

In previous chapters, and in Table 7, it was indicated that females have a lower maximal oxygen uptake capacity when compared to males, at the age of 10 to 12 years and older. Prior to 10 to 12 years of age, the values for males and females are nearly identical. Several factors have been suggested as the primary explanation for these differences. First, the female has a smaller stroke volume than the male for the same absolute level of work, which is at least partially related to her smaller body size. In addition, hemoglobin levels in females have been reported to be lower than males of similar age by as much as 10% or more. With a smaller stroke volume at maximum work, and a similar maximum heart rate, the maximum cardiac output will be lower in the female, and when this is combined with lower hemoglobin levels, the oxygen-carrying and oxygen-delivering capability of the female is greatly reduced. Theoretically, this explains the lower maximal oxygen uptake values in females.

In studies of highly conditioned women distance runners, however, the magnitude of difference when compared to equally trained men distance runners was less, *i.e.,* approximately 16%. In fact, when the best women runners were compared to the best men runners, the differences in maximal oxygen uptake were reduced to only 4.1%. From these results, it would appear that the average female has a tremendous potential for developing her cardiorespiratory endurance capacity to a level far in excess of her existing level. Optimal development of cardiorespiratory endurance capacity would be particularly beneficial for the female athlete, particularly if she is an endurance athlete.

Menstrual and Gynecological Considerations

Two questions which are foremost in the minds of many women, particularly women athletes, have to do with the influence of their menstrual cycle on athletic performance, and the influence of their training procedures and competition on menstruation and childbirth. With respect to alterations in athletic performance ability with different phases of the menstrual cycle, there appears to be a considerable amount of individual variability. Some women have absolutely no noticeable change in their ability to perform throughout the complete cycle, while others have considerable difficulty in the pre-flow and initial-flow phases of the cycle. The limited research which has been conducted tends to suggest that performance ability appears to be best in the immediate post-flow period up to the fifteenth day of the cycle, with the first day of the cycle corresponding to the initiation of the flow or menstrual phase, with ovulation occuring on about day fourteen. The number of women who report impaired performance during the flow phase is approximately the same as those who experience no difficulty. In fact, some women athletes have noted improved performance during the flow phase, including the setting of world records.

With respect to the question concerning the influence of various training procedures and intense competition on the menstrual cycle and childbirth, again, the data is very limited. Several long-term studies have been reported on former competitive swimmers, with findings that suggest that intense training at an early age has no serious consequences relative to future gynecological problems or problems with childbirth. It is generally accepted that the woman who is in excellent physical condition during pregnancy will have an easier period of labor, and fewer undesirable side effects during the actual delivery. With respect to the continuation of an exercise program during pregnancy, this is generally advisable and should be encouraged, providing the supervising physician is in agreement, and that there are no signs of complications. As the expectant mother reaches the last trimester, she will probably have to reduce the intensity of exercise, and possibly even the duration, due to the increasing size of the fetus. This will depend a great deal, however, on the individual and the situation.

One possible problem has surfaced recently, although it is possibly not a problem but a very natural response of the body. Athletes who have trained and competed intensely in sports such as figure skating, dancing, gymnastics, cycling, and distance running have reported the absence of menses or menstrual periods for intervals of months or even years. This absence of menstrual periods or the cessation of menstruation is referred to as *secondary amenorrhea*. Oligomenorrhea, or abnormally infrequent or scanty menses, is also an associated occurrence. The actual percentage of women athletes who experience secondary amenorrhea or oligomenorrhea is not well documented, with estimates of from 4% to 12% on the low end, up to 50% on the high end. The actual percentage of women involved will probably vary according to the sport and to the intensity of training. The occurrence appears to be greater in those who are doing many hours of training each day—*e.g.*, dancers and gymnasts—and to those who are working at high intensities, *e.g.*, distance runners and cyclists. Many of these athletes are thankful to be rid of the "curse," but many are also concerned about the long-term consequences. Neither the cause of secondary amenorrhea or oligomenorrhea, nor the long-term consequences are known. Some of these athletes have become pregnant during the interval of amenorrhea, which is indicative of the fact that fertility is possibly not influenced in the absence of menstruation. This latter point is an important one, for many assume that this is an effective method of birth control, and that they are safe during these intervals of cessation of menstruation. The cause may be related to low levels of weight or body fat, to the acute effects of stress, or to levels of circulating hormones. Research is presently in progress to look both at cause and long-term consequences.

EXERCISE AND AGING

Figure 18 in Chapter 3 is an excellent summary of the relationship between exercise and aging. From this figure it is clear that aging is inevitable. However, equally clear is the fact that by maintaining moderate to high levels of physical conditioning, the individual can have the physiological capacity of the average man or woman who is 20 to 30 years younger! There is ample evidence now that the continuation of vigorous exercise throughout life will reduce the rate of decline in the basic physiological function of the body. What changes in body function take place as one ages?

First, the basal metabolic rate (BMR) decreases at a rate of approximately 3% per decade, starting from the age of 3 through old age to death. Up to the age of 20 to 30 years, this decreased BMR is assumed to be a reflection of a more efficient body metabolism. Beyond the age of 30 years, this decrease is thought to reflect a decrease in the lean body tissue, primarily muscle mass. A decrease in BMR indicates that there will also be a decrease in the total calories that will be necessary each day to provide the energy needs of the individual. Lung function appears to be markedly altered with age. With respect to pulmonary function, vital capacity, and that fraction of the vital capacity which can be exhaled during the first second of a maximal forced expiration, in addition to the forced, expiratory flow rate, all demonstrate a linear decrease with age, starting at between 20 and 30 years of age. The residual lung volume increases, and the total lung capacity remains unchanged. These changes are consistent with the reduced maximal ventilatory capacity with age in exhaustive exercise. Each of these changes indicates a reduced efficiency and capacity of the lungs, and is the result of a loss of elasticity of the lung tissue and the chest wall. The decrease in mobility of the chest wall with aging is thought to be the major cause of the reduction in lung functions.

A number of changes occur in cardiovascular function with aging. As was mentioned earlier, there is a decrease in maximal heart rate with age. Cross-sectional studies estimate the decreases to be approximately a 1-beat-per-minute decrease each year. Recent longitudinal studies indicate that the cross-sectional estimates may be too high. Their data suggest a decrease of only one-half of a beat per minute each year. Maximum stroke volume and maximum cardiac output decrease with age, as does the capacity for peripheral blood flow. However, it is difficult to determine how much of this decrease is due to true aging, and how much is the result of an increasingly sedentary life-style. Heart weight and heart volume increase with aging, while blood volume and total hemoglobin levels tend to stay the same.

The maximal oxygen uptake decreases with age, as was mentioned above and illustrated in Figure 18. Peak maximal oxygen uptake values are obtained between the ages of 17 and 25 years in the male, and between 10 and 13 years in the female. The earlier onset of decline in the female is attributed to her increasingly sedentary life-style once she reaches puberty. The decrease in maximal oxygen uptake with aging is partially the result of a reduced activity level, but the reduction will occur even in those who maintain themselves in peak physical condition. This decrease which occurs irrespective of activity levels is probably the result of a reduction in stroke volume and cardiac output, although the decrease in pulmonary ventilation and a decrease in maximum diffusion capacity may also be contributing factors.

Muscular strength demonstrates a linear decrease with age starting sometime between the ages of 30 and 40 years. By 60 years of age the male has not lost more than 10% to 20% of his peak maximum strength. This loss in strength is the result of inactivity as well as basic changes in the structure of muscle, which include a loss of protein due to alterations in protein synthesis.

When individuals 60 years of age and older initiate a program of exercise, the alterations in physiological function which they will experience will be similar to those experienced by individuals of a much younger age. The major difference in response to training between the younger and the older individual is in magnitude, *i.e.*, the older individual does not respond or adapt to the same extent. Nonetheless, studies have shown that the individual is able to function much more efficiently in performing his daily activities.

Will vigorous exercise pursued throughout one's lifetime provide him with a guarantee of a longer life span? At this point in time, research data is not available to answer that question. Some have made the statement that a lifetime of vigorous exercise may not improve the quantity of life, but it certainly does improve the quality of life. While the research data is presently lacking, most scientists and clinicians who have studied this problem seriously feel that it will only be a matter of time until evidence becomes available to indicate that the quantity of life is also increased. Until that time, most of these individuals continue their programs of vigorous activity.

11

Proper Nutrition for Exercise and Sport

INTRODUCTION

During the 1970s nutrition became one of the most popular topics of magazine articles, books, newspaper columns, and debate! The old adage, "Never discuss or debate politics and religion," should be modified to: "Never discuss or debate politics, religion, and *nutrition*!" The field of nutrition is one of extreme contrasts. On the one side are the self-proclaimed experts who have all of the answers, and on the other side are those who are truly students of nutrition who realize that the field is short on fact and long on fiction and myths. The science of nutrition has advanced considerably over the past decade, but there is still far more to be learned than is presently available. The American public is hungry for information on nutrition, and consequently, frequently falls prey to the latest fad, whether it be a new diet or a new use for an old vitamin. The gullibility of the American public in nutrition and related areas is almost beyond belief. Literally billions of dollars are spent each year as the public experiments with the latest book or gimmick on the market. In 1973, it was estimated that over $10,000,000,000 was being spent each year in the diet industry alone. Over $1,000,000,000 was spent on special diet food. *Dr. Atkins' Diet Revolution* sold approximately 1,000,000 copies in 7 months, and Dr. Stillman's *Quick Weight Loss Diet* sold approximately 5,000,000 copies in 6 years. Over $54,000,000 was spent on "legal" diet pills alone. With the public so willing to part with its money, it is no wonder that so many charlatans have descended to grab a "piece of the action." The average consumer must be better educated and aware of the tremendous potential for fraud, misrepresentation, and misguided zeal.

The present chapter is intended to provide sound information in a highly controversial area. The major focus will be on nutrition as it relates to health, fitness, and sport. The first section will discuss the basic foundation of proper nutrition, and the second section will investigate the role of nutrition in exercise and sport. For more detailed information, a series of excellent books has been listed in the appendix under Selected Readings.

GENERAL CONCEPTS IN NUTRITION

Food is composed of 6 major components: water, minerals, vitamins, proteins, fats, and carbohydrates. Each of these components is an essential ingredient in the daily diet, and has specific functions to perform to maintain the body's health equilibrium. A brief discussion of these components will allow a better understanding of the nature, importance, major sources, and recommended levels of daily intake for each.

Water

Seldom is water thought of as a food. However, it is, in many respects, the most essential of the 6 nutrients. An individual can go for weeks and even months without food, but man can survive without water only for a matter of a few days. Next to oxygen, it is the most important constituent for the maintenance of life. Man can lose most of his fat and carbohydrate stores, and half of his protein, with up to a 40-pound loss of body weight, and survive, but a 20% loss of body water may result in death, and severe disorders occur with a loss of only 10%.

Water is a solvent in which all metabolic changes take place. It functions in digestion, absorption, circulation, and excretion. It assists in two very important regulatory functions: electrolyte balance and regulation of body temperature. In addition, water constitutes from 50% to 70% of the total body weight. Water is supplied from three major sources: fluids, foods, and metabolism. While fluid intake constitutes the major source of water (1.0 to 2.0 liters per day), a substantial amount of water is contained in food. Water constitutes 94% to 96% of lettuce, 95% of radishes, sour pickles, and celery, and 88% of an orange, as examples of a few selected foods. When food is metabolized in the body, water is an important by-product. For every 100 grams of fat, carbohydrate, or protein metabolized, the net yield of "metabolic" water is 107, 55, and 41 grams, respectively. Finally, water is eliminated from the body through the kidneys as urine, through the intestines as feces, through the skin as sweat, and through the lungs as water vapor.

Water needs will vary considerably from day to day depending on a number of factors. Two of the biggest sources of fluctuation in water needs are exercise and either or both high temperature and humidity. These were discussed in considerable detail in Chapter 9. The major problem associated with a lack of water is dehydration, and dehydration should be avoided at all costs. It is a wise practice to consume slightly more water each day than is required by the mechanisms which control thirst. This will assure proper hydration, and any excess water will be passed off in the urine.

Minerals

Minerals have been defined nutritionally as the inorganic elements found in the body. While the body contains more than 20 minerals, approximately 17 have been proved essential in the diet. Minerals of the body are classified into two groups: those present in relatively large amounts, and those needed in very small amounts. This latter group is referred to as the trace minerals. Those present in large amounts include sodium, potassium, calcium, phosphorus, magnesium, sulfur, and various chlorides. Of these, calcium and phosphorus in the teeth and bones account for 60% to 85% of all minerals in the body. The trace minerals include iron, zinc, selenium, manganese, iodine, copper, fluorine, and chromium.

A well-balanced diet which supplies at least 1,500 calories is typically sufficient to provide all of the body's needs for the essential minerals. With heavy exercise, several of the key minerals are lost in abundant quantities, *e.g.*, sodium cloride in sweat; however, the subsequent increase in food intake is more than sufficient to make up for these losses. Iron is the one trace mineral of which a rather sizable percentage of the population have deficiencies. Scientists have estimated that from 20% to 25% of the world's population may be deficient in iron.

Those minerals of greatest importance to body function are listed in Table 21 (pages 196-197). For each mineral listed, there is a description of the location within the body where the mineral is found, the major function of the mineral, and the best food sources for obtaining the mineral in the diet.

Vitamins

Vitamins are a group of unrelated organic compounds needed only in extremely small quantities in the diet, but essential for specific metabolic reactions within the cell, and for normal growth and maintenance of health. Vitamins were relatively unknown until the beginning of the century. Subsequently, approximately 20 vitamins have been identified, and several more have been postulated. Vitamins fall into two basic categories: those which are fat-soluble, and those which are water-

TABLE 21. Mineral elements in the body

MINERAL	PRIMARY LOCATION IN BODY	PRIMARY FUNCTION	FOOD SOURCES
Calcium	bones and teeth	blood clotting, bone formation, transportation of fluids, muscle contraction	milk and milk products, broccoli, sardines, clams, and oysters
Phosphorus	bones and teeth	bone formation, body's energy system, pH regulation	cheese, egg yolk, milk, meat, fish, poultry, whole-grain cereals, legumes, and nuts
Magnesium	bone and inside cells	activates enzymes	whole-grain cereals, nuts, meat, milk, green vegetables, and legumes
Sodium	bone and extra-cellular fluid	regulation of body fluid osmolarity, pH, and body fluid volume	table salt, seafood, milk, and eggs, although abundant in most food except fruits
Chlorine	extracellular fluid	buffer and enzyme activation	table salt, seafood, milk, meat, and eggs
Potassium	intracellular fluid	regulation of body fluid osmolarity, pH, and cell membrane transfer	fruits, meat, milk, cereals, vegetables, and legumes
Sulfur	amino acids	oxidation-reduction reactions	protein foods including meat, fish, poultry, eggs, milk, cheese, legumes, and nuts
Iron	hemoglobin, liver, spleen, and bone	oxygen transportation	liver, meat, egg yolk, legumes, whole or enriched grains, dark green vegetables, shrimp, oysters
Zinc	most tissues, with higher amounts in liver, muscle, and bone	constituent of essential enzymes and insulin	milk, liver, shellfish, herring, and wheat bran
Copper	all tissues, with larger amounts in the liver, brain, heart, and kidney	constituent of enzymes	liver, shellfish, whole grains, cherries, legumes, kidney, poultry, oysters, chocolate, and nuts
Iodine	thyroid gland	essential constituent of thyroxin	iodized table salt, seafood, water, and vegetables
Manganese	bone, pituitary, liver, pancreas, and gastro-intestinal tissue	constituent of essential enzymes	grains, nuts, legumes, fruit, and tea
Fluorine	bone	reduces dental caries and may reduce bone loss	drinking water, tea, coffee, soybeans, spinach, gelatin, onions, and lettuce

TABLE 21. Mineral elements in the body (continued)

MINERAL	PRIMARY LOCATION IN BODY	PRIMARY FUNCTION	FOOD SOURCES
Molybdenum	enzymes	constituent of essential enzymes	legumes, cereal grains, dark green leafy vegetables, and organs
Cobalt	in all cells	essential to normal function of all cells	liver, kidney, oysters, clams, poultry, and milk
Selenium	the cell	fat metabolism	grains, onions, meats, milk, and vegetables
Chromium	the cell	glucose metabolism	corn oil, clams, whole-grain cereals, meat, and drinking water

soluble. Vitamins A, D, E, and K are soluble in fat, while vitamins C and the B-complex vitamins are water-soluble. A fat-soluble vitamin can be stored in the liver and in the fatty tissues of the body. This is an extremely important point, for vitamin toxicity can occur when the body consumes too much of a specific fat-soluble vitamin over long periods of time. Vitamins A and D have been shown to be the most common of the fat-soluble vitamins to exhibit significant impairment of bodily function with toxicity. Water-soluble vitamins are soluble in water, and, as such, they cannot be stored in the body, and any excessive intake of these vitamins will only find their way into the urine and out of the body. With an annual consumption of $300,000,000 to $500,000,000 worth of vitamin supplements each year, our country must produce the most expensive urine in the world. Most, if not all, vitamin supplementation is unnecessary. This will be discussed later. The vitamins, their sources and functions, and the problems associated with deficiencies are listed in Table 22 (pages 198-199).

Proteins

Protein was the first substance recognized as a vital part of living tissue, and is now known to be the fundamental structural compound of cells, antibodies, enzymes, and many hormones. Most protein is located in muscle tissue, but it is also distributed in the soft tissues, bone, teeth, blood, and other body fluids. Proteins are comprised of at least 23 different amino acids, of which between 8 and 10 are referred to as essential amino acids. The essential amino acids are those which can't be synthesized by the body, and are therefore essential to include in the diet. If there is a shortage or deficiency of any of these essential amino acids, there will be serious limitations placed on growth and general body

TABLE 22. Vitamins and their functions, sources, and associated deficiency states

VITAMIN	PRIMARY FUNCTION	SOURCES	DEFICIENCY STATES
	FAT-SOLUBLE VITAMINS		
A	adaptation to dim light, resistance to infection, prevents eye and skin disorders, bone and tooth development	liver, kidney, milk, butter, egg yolk, yellow vegetables, apricots, cantaloupe, and peaches	night blindness
D	facilitates absorption of calcium; bone and tooth development	sunlight, fish, eggs, fortified dairy products, and liver	rickets
E	prevents oxidation of essential vitamins and fatty acids and protects red blood cells from hemolysis	wheatgerm, vegetable oils, green vegetables, milk fat, egg yolk, and nuts	no known at this time
K	blood clotting	liver, soybean oil, vegetable oil, green vegetables, tomatoes, cauliflower, and wheat bran	hemorrhage disease
	WATER-SOLUBLE VITAMINS		
B_1 (thiamine)	energy metabolism, growth, appetite, and digestion	pork, liver, organs, meat, legumes, whole-grain enriched cereals and breads, wheatgerm, and potatoes	beriberi
B_2 (riboflavin)	growth, health of eyes, and energy metabolism	milk and dairy foods, organ meats, green vegetables, eggs, fish, and enriched cereals and breads	mouth and lip lesions, loss of vision
Niacin	energy metabolism and fatty acid synthesis	fish, liver, meat, poultry, grains, eggs, peanuts, milk, and legumes	pellagra, limited energy production
B_6 (pyridoxine)	protein metabolism and growth	pork, glandular meats, cereal bran and germ, milk, egg yolk, oatmeal, and legumes	convulsions, anemia
Pantothenic acid	hemoglobin formation, and carbohydrate, protein, and fat metabolism	whole-grain cereals, organ meats, and eggs	no known at this time
Biotin	carbohydrate, fat, and protein metabolism	liver, peanuts, yeast, milk, meat, egg yolk, cereal, nuts, legumes, bananas, grapefruit, tomatoes, watermelon, and strawberries	no known at this time
Folic acid (folacin)	growth, fat metabolism, maturation of red blood cells	green vegetables, organ meats, lean beef, wheat, eggs, fish, dry beans, lentils, asparagus, broccoli, and yeast	anemia

TABLE 22. Vitamins and their functions, sources and associated deficiency states (continued)

VITAMIN	PRIMARY FUNCTION	SOURCES	DEFICIENCY STATES
B$_{12}$ (cobalamin)	red blood cell production, nervous system metabolism, and fat metabolism	liver, kidney, milk and dairy foods, and meat	anemia, neuromuscular weakness
C (ascorbic acid)	growth, tissue repair, tooth and bone formation	citrus fruits, tomatoes, strawberries, potatoes, melons, peppers, and pineapple	scurvy

function. Proteins are derived from both animal tissue and from the seeds, or grains, of plants. Those who are on vegetarian, or modified vegetarian, diets will be able to obtain the essential amino acids providing their food choices are selected carefully. A lacto-vegetarian diet (includes milk and milk products) or a lacto-ovo-vegetarian diet (includes eggs as well as milk and milk products) provides an even greater opportunity for meeting the basic requirements for protein as well as the other essential nutrients.

Proteins serve many critical functions in the body. They are used in repairing tissue which has become worn out from constant use, as well as in building new tissue. The amino acids are considered to be the building blocks of tissue, and protein is their only source. Proteins are involved in almost all body secretions and fluids, including enzymes, some hormones, mucus, milk, and sperm. Proteins also are important in the body's osmotic reactions which control fluid volumes, in the body's resistance to disease through antibodies, and in the body's blood-clotting mechanism. Finally, hemoglobin, which is the oxygen carrier in the blood, is composed of iron (heme) and a large protein molecule (globin).

Approximately 5% to 15% of the total calories ingested per day are from protein. It has been estimated that the average American consumes between two and three times the total amount of protein that he needs. This excess is totally unnecessary, expensive, and is potentially harmful. The daily recommended allowances published in 1980 by the National Research Council for the average man and woman are 56 and 44 grams of protein per day, respectively, which are reduced from the 1968 recommendations of 65 and 55 grams per day. These recommendations are for the average-sized person, *i.e.,* a 70-kilogram (154-pound) man and a 55-kilogram (120-pound) woman. The recommended intake would be increased or decreased proportionally depending on body weight. For the mature adult, an allowance of approximately 0.8 grams per kilogram of body weight is considered appropriate.

Fats

Fats or lipids are terms used to define a similar group of compounds which are insoluble in water, soluble in organic solvents such as ether and chloroform, and utilizable by living organisms. A fat consists of two different clusters of atoms: glycerol and fatty acid. When glycerol and fatty acid molecules are bound chemically, they form triglycerides. Most natural fats are composed of between 98% and 99% triglyceride. Lipids are generally classified into one of three categories: simple, compound, and derived. Simple lipids include fatty acids, neutral fats (including triglycerides), and waxes. Compound lipids include phospholipids, glycolipids, and lipoproteins. Derived lipids include mono- and di-glycerides, glycerol, sterols (including cholesterol), and fat-soluble vita-mins. Chapters 1 and 2 included a detailed discussion of cholesterol and its relationship to coronary artery disease, with specific reference to the lipoprotein carriers of cholesterol.

There are two types of fatty acids: saturated and unsaturated. The difference between the two is in the bonding between carbon and hydro-gen atoms. Unsaturated fats contain one (monounsaturated) or more (polyunsaturated) double bonds between carbon atoms in a chain of carbon atoms. Each double bond in the chain takes the place of two hydrogen atoms. When the carbon chain is saturated with hydrogen atoms—*i.e.*, two hydrogen atoms for each carbon atom—this is referred to as a saturated fatty acid. In practical terms, a saturated fat is in the form of a solid, *i.e.*, animal fat, and an unsaturated fat is in the form of a liquid, *i.e.*, fish and vegetable oil. By the process of hydrogenation, unsaturated oils can be changed from a liquid to a semi-solid state. Saturated fats are derived primarily from animal sources, including the fat in meats such as beef, lamb, pork, and chicken, and in egg and dairy products such as egg yolk, milk, cream, and cheese. Unsaturated fats are derived primarily from plant sources.

Fat is an extremely important energy source both at rest and during light to moderate exercise. Fats are the most concentrated source of food energy in the diet, providing over twice the number of calories per unit of weight than either carbohydrates or proteins. Fat is also easily stored, and is a ready source of energy under almost all conditions. Fat is the only source of linoleic acid, and is the mode of transportation in the body for the fat-soluble vitamins. Fat plays an important part in the regulation of body temperature, since it is an excellent insulator. While this works to the advantage of the individual in cold weather, it is a distinct disadvan-tage during the hot weather months. Fat also serves to protect the vital organs such as the heart, liver, kidneys, spleen, brain, and spinal cord. Finally, fat adds palatability to food, and due to its slow passage from the stomach it tends to satiate the appetite, or reduce the feeling of hunger, for longer periods of time.

Fat constitutes approximately 45% of the total calories consumed in the diet of the average American, which is a considerably higher percentage of fat intake compared to that at the turn of this century. Current recommendations suggest that fat should constitute only 25% to 30% of our total calories, and that the reductions in fat intake should come from saturated fats. There is presently a great deal of controversy on specific recommendations for the intake of saturated fats, particularly in reference to egg and dairy products as they relate to coronary artery disease.

Carbohydrates

Carbohydrates are represented by the various sugars and starches, and are the most efficient, and usually the least expensive, source of food energy. They are classified as monosaccharides, disaccharides, and polysaccharides. Glucose, fructose, galactose, and mannose are the monosaccharides, or simple sugars. Disaccharides are double sugars, or the bonding of two simple monosaccharides, and are exemplified by sucrose (glucose and fructose), maltose (glucose and glucose), and lactose (glucose and galactose). Sucrose is ordinary table sugar and is found mainly in sugar cane and sugar beets. Polysaccharides are composed of three or more monosaccharides and include starch and glycogen. Glycogen is the form in which glucose is stored in the body. The term *glycogenosis* refers to the process of transforming glucose to glycogen, while *glycogenolysis* refers to the breakdown of glycogen to glucose in the liver.

In addition to being a ready energy source, which is particularly important as a fuel source for high-intensity exercise, carbohydrates also exert an influence on both protein and fat metabolism, sparing the use of protein as an energy source, and controlling the amount of fat that is utilized. Glucose is critical as the sole energy source for the brain and is essential for maintenance of the functional integrity of the nervous system.

Carbohydrates constitute approximately 50% to 60% of the total dietary calories consumed by the average American, but this percentage has been decreasing since the early 1900s. This decrease has come from a decreased intake of starches, for the intake of sugars has actually increased. The major sources of sugars and starches are grains, fruits, vegetables, milk, and concentrated sweets. Refined sugar, syrup, and cornstarch are examples of pure carbohydrates, and many of the concentrated sweets such as candy, honey, jellies, molasses, and soft drinks contain few, if any, other nutrients. These have been referred to as "empty calories" since they contribute nothing but calories to the diet.

Recommended Dietary Allowances

In the 1940s, the potential for nutrition-related health problems was recognized and the Food and Nutrition Board of the National Research Council of the National Academy of Sciences was formed and published the first report known as the *Recommended Dietary Allowances,* or RDA. These original recommendations are revised periodically, and they are intended to provide guidelines for planning and evaluating food intake. These recommended allowances are specified for total energy intake, and for protein, vitamin, and mineral intake. The recommendations are based on the age and sex of the individual, and include the special circumstances of pregnant and lactating women. The 1980 RDA's are provided in Table 23 (page 203). With the new practice of labeling the nutrient contents of

TABLE 23. Recommended Daily Dietary Allowances,[a] 1980. From the Food and Nutrition Board, National Research Council of the National Academy of Sciences

Designed for the maintenance of good nutrition of practically all healthy people in the U.S.A.

	Age	Weight		Height		Energy	Protein	Vita-min A Activity		Vita-min D	Vita-min E Activity[c]
	(years)	(kg)	(lbs)	(cm)	(in)	(kcal)[b]	(g)	(RE)[f]	(IV)	(IV)	(IV)
Infants	0.0-0.5	6	13	60	24	kg×115	kg×2.2	420[d]	1,400	400	3
	0.5-1.0	9	20	71	28	kg×105	kg×2.0	400	2,000	400	4
Children	1-3	13	29	90	35	1,300	23	400	2,000	400	5
	4-6	20	44	112	44	1,700	30	500	2,500	400	6
	7-10	28	62	132	52	2,400	34	700	3,300	400	7
Males	11-14	45	99	157	62	2,700	45	1,000	5,000	400	8
	15-18	66	145	176	70	2,800	56	1,000	5,000	400	10
	19-22	70	154	177	70	2,900	56	1,000	5,000	300	10
	23-50	70	154	178	70	2,700	56	1,000	5,000	200	10
	51+	70	154	178	70	2,400	56	1,000	5,000	200	10
Females	11-14	46	101	157	62	2,200	46	800	4,000	400	8
	15-18	55	120	163	64	2,100	46	800	4,000	400	8
	19-22	55	120	163	64	2,100	44	800	4,000	400	8
	23-50	55	120	163	64	2,000	44	800	4,000	200	8
	51+	55	120	163	64	1,800	44	800	4,000	200	8
Pregnant						+300	+30	+200	+1,000	+200	+2
Lactating						+500	+20	+400	+2,000	+200	+3

[a]The allowances are intended to provide for individual variations among most normal persons as they live in the United States under usual environmental stresses. Diets should be based on a variety of common foods in order to provide other nutrients for which human requirements have been less well defined.

[b]Kilojoules (kJ)—4.2 × kcal.

[c]Retinol equivalents.

most packaged foods, these RDA's have much more meaning and significance. Still, the numbers and unfamiliar units of measure make these recommendations of limited value for most individuals, and eventually led the Department of Agriculture to create and publish a simplified plan, titled "The Essentials of an Adequate Diet."

This publication provided a much more simplified approach to diet and menu planning. The "Four-Food-Group Plan" establishes recommendations for daily food intake in each of four basic areas: milk and milk products; meat and high-protein foods; fruits and vegetables; and cereals and grain foods. Table 24 (page 204) outlines the "Four-Food-Group Plan," including the number of servings per day and the major contributions of each food group. It should be emphasized that these recommendations are based on meeting the minimal requirements, and will have to be increased either by larger or more servings for individuals who are active and expend a considerable amount of additional energy each day. The individual with a weight problem, however, should take a close look at Table 23 to determine if the total number of calories taken in each day exceeds the RDA for sex, weight, and age. If a reduction in calories is

WATER-SOLUBLE VITAMINS							MINERALS					
Acorbic Acid (mg)	Folacin$f$ (μg)	Niacin (mg)	Riboflavin (mg)	Thiamin (mg)	Vitamin B$_6$ (mg)	Vitamin B$_{12}$ (μg)	Calcium (mg)	Phosphorus (mg)	Iodine (μg)	Iron (mg)	Magnesium (mg)	Zinc (mg)
35	30	6	0.4	0.3	0.3	0.5	360	240	40	10	50	3
35	45	8	0.6	0.5	0.6	1.5	540	360	50	15	70	5
45	100	9	0.8	0.7	0.9	2.0	800	800	70	15	150	10
45	200	11	1.0	0.9	1.3	2.5	800	800	90	10	200	10
45	300	16	1.4	1.2	1.6	3.0	800	800	120	10	250	10
50	400	18	1.6	1.4	1.8	3.0	1,200	1,200	150	18	350	15
60	400	18	1.7	1.4	2.0	3.0	1,200	1,200	150	18	400	15
60	400	19	1.7	1.5	2.2	3.0	800	800	150	10	350	15
60	400	18	1.6	1.4	2.2	3.0	800	800	150	10	350	15
60	400	16	1.4	1.2	2.2	3.0	800	800	150	10	350	15
50	400	15	1.3	1.1	1.8	3.0	1,200	1,200	150	18	300	15
60	400	14	1.3	1.1	2.0	3.0	1,200	1,200	150	18	300	15
60	400	14	1.3	1.1	2.0	3.0	800	800	150	18	300	15
60	400	13	1.2	1.0	2.0	3.0	800	800	150	18	300	15
60	400	13	1.2	1.0	2.0	3.0	800	800	150	10	300	15
+20	+400	+2	+0.3	+0.4	+0.6	+1.0	+400	+400	+25	30	+150	+5
+40	+100	+5	+0.5	+0.5	+0.5	+1.0	+400	+400	+50	+30	+150	+10

dAssumed to be all as retinol in milk during the first six months of life. All subsequent intakes are assumed to be half as retinol and half as β-carotene when calculated from international units. As retinol equivalents, three fourths are as retinol and one fourth as β-carotene.

eTotal vitamin E activity, estimated to be 80 percent as α-tocopherol and 20 percent other tocopherols. See text for variation in allowances.

fThe folacin allowances refer to dietary sources as determined by *Lactobacillus casei* assay. Pure forms of folacin may be effective in doses less than one fourth of the recommended dietary allowance.

TABLE 24. The basic "Four-Food-Group Plan"

FOOD GROUP	DAILY AMOUNTS FOR ADULTS	NUTRITIONAL CONTRIBUTION
Milk and Milk Products	Two or more servings per day either as a milk beverage or a milk product such as cheese and ice cream; a serving would be one cup or its equivalent	Protein Calcium Riboflavin Vitamin D
Meat and High-Protein Products	Two or more servings of meat, fish, poultry, eggs, or vegetables such as dried beans, lentils, peas, and nuts; a serving of meat, fish, or poultry would be 3.5 ounces of lean and boneless meat	Protein Thiamin Iron Niacin Riboflavin
Fruits and Vegetables	Four or more servings per day of ½ cup or more	Vitamin A Vitamin C Folic acid
Cereals and Grains	Four or more servings per day with one serving equal to one slice of bread, ½ to ¾ cup of cooked cereal, macaroni, spaghetti, etc.	Protein Thiamin Riboflavin Niacin Iron

recommended, this should be accomplished by reducing the size of the servings in all food groups and not by reducing the number of servings in any one group. A balanced diet is the goal or objective for the total population, and should include approximately 10% to 15% protein, 30% to 35% fat, and 50% to 60% carbohydrate, minimizing saturated fat and concentrated sugars.

Dietary Supplements

The food industry makes a considerable amount of money each year in the area of dietary supplements. Is there a need for vitamin and mineral supplementation? What advantages are to be gained from protein supplementation? It would appear that for the individual who is getting a well-balanced diet, and is moderately active, dietary supplementation is totally unnecessary. This is a highly controversial area, for literally thousands of people can give personal testimonies as to how much help they received and how much better they feel from supplementing one or more of the vitamins. It is difficult, if not impossible, to refute these claims. However, the basic research which is highly controlled to avoid personal biases would indicate that such claims are unfounded. This is not to deny that some good may have been achieved in some individuals, but the research literature overwhelmingly supports the position that supplements are not necessary. Logically, supplements would not be expected to provide any benefits. With the exception of the fat-soluble vitamins, supplementation of water-soluble vitamins and minerals will not result in any long-term effects since they are rapidly excreted in the urine. Protein is already being consumed in the diet at levels in excess of two to three times that which is needed. Further supplementation of protein will have no additional benefits.

What about the athlete or recreational jogger? Won't their needs for additional vitamins, minerals, and protein be increased as they increase their total caloric expenditure above that of the moderately active individual? In reality, the answer to this question is no. The protein requirement will go up in proportion to the additional energy that is being expended each day, but the increased food intake will more than take care of the increased requirement. The recommendations for most vitamins and minerals are established independent of exercise habits, *i.e.,* increased levels of activity essentially don't alter the basic requirements. In addition, the food intake tends to parallel the level of activity, so the individual who exercises vigorously each day is probably taking in far more vitamins than needed. Supplementation may be necessary, however, for the individual who is on a calorie-restricted diet. When the total calorie intake per day decreases to 1,500 calories or less, there may be need for a general multi-vitamin.

NUTRITION IN EXERCISE AND SPORT

For centuries man has related his success or failure in athletics to what he ate or drank either before or during competition. Mystical qualities have been ascribed to buffalo meat, dessicated liver, bee pollen, fructose, amino acid supplements, honey, and numerous other foods, vitamins, or minerals. Is it possible to manipulate the diet to achieve an improvement in performance? The answer to that question is a qualified yes, although improvement is limited to the manipulation in only one or two nutritional areas, and the degree of improvement is still debatable. Unfortunately, so much of the research that has been conducted in this area has lacked adequate controls. It is appropriate to use the double-blind technique for this type of research, where neither the subject in the study nor the principle scientist or investigator has knowledge as to which group is receiving a certain dietary supplement and which is receiving a placebo. Only after the study has been completed does a third party come forward with the key as to who received what treatment. While this is the most appropriate technique to use, few studies have employed it, which leaves one highly suspicious of those studies which failed to use this technique.

Protein Supplements

As was discussed in detail in the previous section, the average diet in America today contains two to three times more protein than is required on a daily basis. Since the amino acids of protein are the essential building blocks for the growth and development of body tissue, it has been the tradition over the years to liberally supplement protein when attempting to achieve increases in muscle bulk and strength through intensive strength training programs. Will this additional supplementation, over and above the excess protein in the normal diet, substantially increase muscle bulk? Logic, and most nutritionists, would answer an emphatic no! However, several recent studies indicate the protein supplementation may increase body protein stores and muscle mass. In one study, two groups of young men were engaged in heavy physical activity and consuming either 1.4 or 2.8 grams of protein per day for every kilogram of body weight for a period of 40 days. The group receiving the increased level of protein did have substantially greater gains in muscle mass and body protein storage. Additional studies investigating the influence of anabolic steroids in promoting gains in muscular strength and size found that the steroids were ineffective unless they were accompanied by a protein supplement. It would appear that protein supplementation may facilitate the growth of muscle, although the gains are not considerable, and probably do not justify the tremendous expense associated with the commercial supplements.

Fat and Carbohydrate

While at one time carbohydrate was considered the primary, if not the only, fuel for muscular exercise, it is now recognized that the role of fat as a primary energy source during exercise is considerable. Fat is essentially an inexhaustible source of fuel, while carbohydrate stores are greatly limited, providing for not more than 60 to 120 minutes of moderately heavy exercise. Since the supply of carbohydrate is limited, it would facilitate performance if either or both carbohydrate stores could be increased, or if fat could be utilized in place of carbohydrate, sparing carbohydrate stores, and theoretically prolonging endurance exercise.

With this in mind, Scandinavian researchers in the 1960s experimented with various combinations of diet and endurance performance. In one study, the subjects were placed on a specific dietary regimen for 3-day intervals and tested on an all-out ride to exhaustion on a bicycle ergometer at a work load that represented 75% of the individual's capacity, *i.e.*, maximal oxygen uptake. The total work time on the bicycle was directly related to the glycogen content in the exercising muscles, and the glycogen content varied in direct response to the diet. After a normal mixed diet, the subjects worked for nearly 126 minutes before they reached exhaustion, and the initial glycogen content in the exercising muscles was 1.93 grams per 100 grams of wet tissue. After 3 days on a diet of fat and protein, with very limited carbohydrate, the subjects' initial glycogen content was 0.69 grams per 100 grams of wet tissue, and the riding time to exhaustion was reduced to only 59 minutes. After an additional 3 days on a high-carbohydrate diet, the subjects started the ride with a glycogen content of 3.70 grams per 100 grams of wet tissue, and were able to prolong the time to exhaustion for the same intensity of exercise to 189 minutes, an improvement of approximately 50% above that for the normal diet, and more than a threefold increase over the high-fat and high-protein diet.

These findings were not totally unexpected, however, since earlier work had shown that exhaustion from endurance exercise was accompanied by hypoglycemia, or low blood sugar, and by low, if not totally depleted, glycogen stores in the active muscle groups. Subsequent studies have verified this rather remarkable response to nutritional manipulation. In one study, the subjects participated in two 30-kilometer cross-country running races, one after a normal mixed diet, and the other following several days on an extremely high-carbohydrate diet. The high-carbohydrate diet resulted in initial muscle glycogen levels that were nearly double the levels attained following the mixed diet, and in substantially improved race times, with the improvement coming essentially in the last half of the race.

This elevation of glycogen stores through nutritional manipulation has been referred to as carbohydrate loading. Subsequent research and self-experimentation by the athletes themselves have refined the carbohydrate loading technique. The athlete must totally deplete his carbohydrate stores approximately 7 to 8 days prior to the day of competition by a high-intensity workout of 60 to 120 minutes in duration. This is then followed by 3 to 4 days of reduced activity and a very low-carbohydrate diet. The final 3 to 4 days prior to competition is the time during which the carbohydrate stores are replenished with a very high-carbohydrate diet, and little or no activity. These last few days are the athlete's reward for all of his hard training and that very difficult period when he was restricted to a very low-carbohydrate intake. Some athletes omit the period of low-carbohydrate intake. This is a much easier regimen to follow, and probably doesn't reduce the overall benefits that much. Angina-like symptoms (chest pain) have been noted in several athletes who have attempted carbohydrate loading. It is unclear as to whether this was truly a cardiovascular problem, or if it was a cardiovascular problem, whether it was related to the actual carbohydrate loading. Recognizing the potential for problems, athletes who attempt this nutritional manipulation should proceed with caution.

The second method in which endurance performance might be facilitated is by shifting the primary energy source from carbohydrate to fat, thus sparing the limited carbohydrate for use later in the exercise. At rest and during exercise, the energy source is seldom from a single fuel, but, rather, is a combination of both fat and carbohydrate. As the intensity of exercise shifts from low or moderate levels to high or exhaustive levels, a greater fraction of the energy is derived from carbohydrate. At any given intensity, if the body could be manipulated to use a higher fraction of fat as the energy source, carbohydrates would be spared, and the individual should, theoretically, be able to prolong the length of the exercise period prior to reaching the state of exhaustion. This theory was tested on both animals and humans, and it was found that increasing the levels of free fatty acids in the blood by either heparin or caffeine increased the utilization of fats and spared the limited carbohydrate stores, thereby increasing the capacity for prolonged endurance exercise. The amount of caffeine needed to accomplish this effect is approximately the equivalent of two cups of coffee, ingested 30 to 60 minutes prior to exercise.

Vitamins and Minerals

Numerous research studies have been conducted to determine the benefits, if any, from the supplementation of various vitamins and minerals. There are a number of studies which indicate some improvement in performance with specific vitamin supplementation, but there are nearly an equal number of studies which show essentially no benefits. In reviewing all of these studies, it would appear that several of the B-complex vitamins, and vitamins C and E, may provide limited beneficial effects, but this conclusion is certainly open to debate. If there is improvement from supplementation of these vitamins, the magnitude of improvement would be very small.

The supplementation of minerals, particularly salt in the form of salt tablets, has been advocated for a number of years. With the loss of salt in sweat, it was theorized that supplementation of salt through salt tablets was essential. It is now recognized that the average individual gets sufficient salt in his diet, even in hot and humid weather when the volume of sweat lost per day is increased considerably. One of the basic adaptations the body makes to heat stress is to reduce the salt content of the sweat, thereby conserving salt. A liberal salting of food is now considered to be sufficient for replacing that salt which was lost. Salt tablets are not advocated, for they could promote the retention of water and the loss of potassium, in addition to having potentially dangerous side effects for persons with high blood pressure. Aspartates, which are potassium and magnesium salts of aspartic acid, have been promoted as a beneficial supplement on the basis of their interaction with blood ammonia. Again, studies are nearly evenly divided as to whether supplementation has any value in improving athletic performance.

Pre-Contest Meal

It has been traditional for the athlete to have a thick, juicy steak, baked potato, and salad as the pre-contest meal. It is now recognized that this is probably the worst possible meal the athlete could eat prior to competition. Steak has a relatively high fat content, and fat slows down the total digestive process. With food still in the stomach and intestine during exercise, this sets up a competition for the available blood supply between the gastrointestinal area and the muscles that are involved in competition. Also, the pre-competition tension also tends to slow the digestive processes, and a heavy meal will frequently lead to nausea and vomiting. As a result, more athletes are switching to very light meals 3 to 4 hours prior to competition, and saving their steak for either the night before or the night after competition. Those who practice carbohydrate loading typically have an extremely large dinner the evening before a race. Traditionally, this has included plates of spaghetti, loaves of bread, and much beer and wine. Since most long-distance races are conducted early in the morning to escape the heat of the day, the large meal the night before competition is probably not advisable. It typically leaves the runner feeling very full and uncomfortable, with the need for a large bowel movement, which hopefully can be accomplished prior to the start of the race. This large meal is traditional and enjoyable, but should be moved back 6 to 24 hours, either to the preceding lunch or dinner, respectively.

The use of a liquid pre-contest meal is becoming popular. A liquid diet is palatable, digests relatively easily, leaves the stomach and intestine quickly, provides the essential nutrients, and is less likely to result in nervous indigestion, nausea, vomiting, and abdominal cramps. This would appear to be a wise choice for a pre-contest meal on the basis of that information presently available. However, each athlete has his own personal preferences and beliefs, and to disturb these may have a much greater negative influence than the positive influence of the liquid diet.

For those athletes who are participating in endurance contests which last for several hours or more, there is probably a need to supplement glucose in the fluids they consume for water and electrolyte replacement. After several hours of endurance exercise, the blood sugar levels start to fall. This can be prevented by the addition of small quantities of glucose to the fluid replacement solution, not to exceed 2.5 grams per 100 milliliters of solution. Glucose in excess of this concentration begins to limit the rate at which the solution empties from the stomach. This reduces the rate of fluid replacement, which is highly undesirable, since fluid replacement is the primary concern relative to the health and safety of the athlete.

12

Prevention and Treatment of Athletic Injuries

INTRODUCTION

The competitive athlete, the recreational athlete, and the individual who is exercising to achieve health-related benefits all have something in common. At one time or another, each will experience an athletic, sport, or exercise-related injury. This may be an injury as serious as a skull fracture or direct blow to the kidney, or it may be something as minor as a simple ankle sprain or a blister on the bottom of the foot. Injuries are, at the least, an inconvenience and a distraction from optimal performance, but they can be devastating, ending in permanent disability and death. Like many diseases, most athletic injuries are preventable, providing the proper precautions are taken in advance. This chapter will discuss the various types of injuries that occur as a result of exercise and sport, list the most common medical problems associated with specific sports, present the most appropriate steps for preventing injury, and, finally, discuss the appropriate techniques for the acute treatment of injuries. Since the area of athletic injuries is so vast in scope, this chapter will, by necessity, be limited to a summary of the major points.

TYPES OF ATHLETIC INJURIES

Dr. Thomas Fahey, in his book *What to Do About Athletic Injuries,**
states that there are four basic types of athletic injuries: sudden traumatic injuries; repeated traumatic injuries; overuse injuries; and imbalance

---

Fahey, T. *What to Do About Athletic Injuries,* New York: Butterick Publishing, 1979.

injuries. A quick blow to the side of the head or a fracture of the femur would be classified as sudden traumatic injuries. A knee which is wrenched in one play in the football game and is continuously subjected to trauma on subsequent plays until the player finally has to remove himself from the game is an example of a repeated trauma injury. Overuse injuries are injuries which result from repetitive movements where the individual isn't properly trained for that level of stress, or where improper techniques are used. Tennis elbow and jogger's knee are examples of overuse injuries. Imbalance injuries are the result of postural imbalances, anatomical weaknesses, and overdevelopment of certain muscle groups at the expense of others.

Most injuries fall into one of two categories: exposed wounds, and unexposed wounds. Exposed wounds include abrasions, lacerations, incisions, and puncture wounds. *Abrasions* are those conditions where the skin is abraded or scraped against a rough surface. The outer layers of skin are torn away, exposing numerous capillaries. *Lacerations* are the result of a sharp or pointed object tearing the tissue, giving the wound an appearance of a jagged-edged cavity. *Puncture wounds* involve the direct penetration of the skin and underlying tissues by a sharp-pointed object, such as a spike or cleat on an athletic shoe. *Incisions* are clean cuts which are frequently the result of a direct blow over a sharp or poorly padded bone.

Unexposed wounds, or closed wounds, are those internal injuries in which the outer layer of skin hasn't been penetrated. These wounds include contusions, strains, sprains, dislocations, and fractures. *Contusions* are bruises, and are the result of traumatic blows to the body. Contusions can be relatively minor or superficial in nature, or they can be major, involving deep tissue tears and hemorrhage. The discoloration which appears within 24 to 48 hours is the result of the hemorrhage which forms a hematoma, or blood clot. Most contusions are relatively minor, and if treated immediately will present few, if any, problems other than localized soreness. Major contusions, however, are much more painful and require considerable time to heal. Football players receive contusions of the thigh as a result of a sharp block or tackle. These are typically tender and extremely painful if direct contact is made with them before they have fully healed.

Strains are commonly referred to as muscle pulls, and represent a tear or rip in the muscle itself or the adjacent tissue. Strains may result from simple minute separations of connective tissue and muscle fiber, to a complete avulsion of the tendon from its bony attachment. Strains are most common in the hamstrings group, gastrocnemius, quadriceps group, hip flexors, hip adductor group, the spinalis group of the back, the deltoid, and the rotator cuff group of the shoulder. A snapping sound may be heard when the tissue tears, which is followed immediately by a sharp pain, and loss of function and severe weakness result. Frequently, spasmodic contractions occur, the specific injured area is very tender to the touch, and an indentation or cavity can be felt where the tissues have separated.

Sprains are the result of a traumatic twisting of the joint which results in either stretching or tearing the stabilizing connective tissues, and represent one of the most common, and frequently one of the most disabling, athletic injuries. In some cases, a severe sprain is much more disabling and takes longer to heal than a fracture in the same general area. With sprains, there is injury to the surrounding ligaments, to the articular capsule and synovial membrane, and to the tendons crossing the joint. Blood and synovial fluid leak into the joint cavity, causing swelling, extreme tenderness, and a limited range of motion. The joints which are most vulnerable to sprain include the ankles, knees, shoulders, wrists, and elbows.

Dislocations result when the joint is forced to go beyond its normal anatomical limitations. Subluxations are partial dislocations in which the separation between two articulating bones is incomplete. Luxations are complete dislocations, in which there is complete separation between two articulating bones. With dislocations, there is an immediate loss of limb function, deformity of the joint is almost always apparent, and swelling and tenderness are immediately present.

Fractures are defined as interruptions in the continuity of the bone, and are classified as either simple or compound. A simple fracture involves a break in the bone without breaking through the skin, whereas in a compound fracture, the bone extends through the outer layers of the skin, which then is classified as an external wound. Fractures can be further classified into the categories that follow. *Comminuted fractures* consist of three or more bone fragments at the fracture site. *Depressed fractures* occur in flat bones such as those comprising the skull. *Greenstick fractures* are incomplete breaks in bones that have not yet completed ossification. *Impacted fractures* are those in which long bones telescope one part of the bone on another, resulting from tremedous forces applied through the long axis of the bone. *Longitudinal fractures* are those in which the bone splits along its length. *Multiple fractures* involve a severe break and separation of bone sections. *Oblique fractures* are breaks which occur at an oblique angle to the long axis of the bone. *Serrated fractures* are those in which there are two bony fragments, each having a saw-toothed, sharp-edged fracture line. *Spiral fractures* give the appearance of a spiral, or S-shaped, separation. *Transverse fractures* occur in a straight line, at right angles to the long axis of the bone. *Stress fractures* are hairline breaks in bone which are the result of overuse or sudden trauma. Stress fractures are sometimes missed on the initial diagnosis, only to show up on later X rays. When a stress fracture is suspected, an X ray should be taken several weeks following the initial complaint.

Several other injuries or problems which do not fall under the classification of wounds include muscle soreness, muscle cramps, muscle spasms, tendinitis, bursitis, blisters, bone bruises, shin splints, and chondromalacia patella. *Muscle soreness* was discussed in Chapter 7, and it was mentioned that the specific cause of muscle soreness is still to be determined. Soreness almost always is involved when a muscle or muscle group is exercised above the intensity at which it is normally exercised. *Muscle cramps* may be due to a salt and potassium imbalance in the muscle. *Muscle spasm* is a term used synonymously with muscle cramps. *Tendinitis* is an inflammation of the sheath which covers the tendon, and is frequently the result of overuse. *Bursitis* refers to inflammation of the bursa, which are closed sacs which contain fluid, and are strategically located in areas of the body where friction or shock occur, such as between a tendon and the underlying bone. *Blisters* are usually the result of excessive friction between the skin and some external surface, such as a shoe. The epidermis separates from the dermis and fluid accumulates between the two layers of skin. *Bone bruises* are painful contusions of bone, most typically the bones of the feet. *Shin splints* refer to a sharp pain along the front aspect of the shin bone or tibia, and are probably the result of a lowered arch, irritated membranes, separation of the muscle from the bone, hairline fracture of the bone, or other factors. *Chondromalacia patella* is a very painful, disabling knee injury which is the result of continued irritation and a breaking down of the undersurface of the patella or kneecap. This is a very common complaint among distance runners, and can be traced, in many cases, to running on a sloped surface where the kneecap is forced to take an unnatural path as it moves through the range of motion.

MEDICAL PROBLEMS ASSOCIATED WITH SPECIFIC SPORTS

In a recent book, Dr. John Bergfeld, team physician for the Cleveland Browns professional football team and orthopedic surgeon at the prestigious Cleveland Clinic, listed all of the common medical problems faced by athletes in various sports. This list is presented in Table 25 (pages 216-217), and the problems are categorized as being the result of trauma, overuse, environmental factors, and illness. Figure 26 (page 214) illustrates where on the body these specific injuries occur. While this list highlights only the major medical problems associated with each sport, it does provide an excellent brief overview.

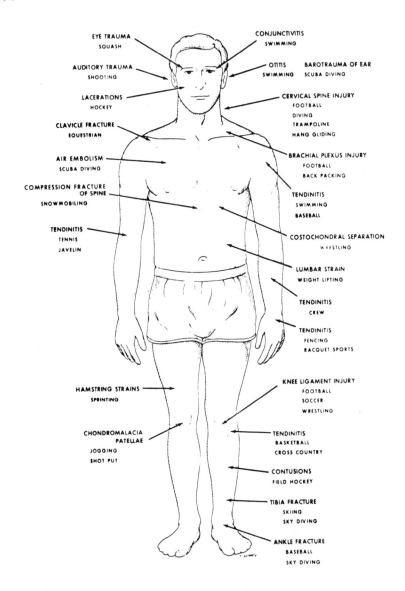

FIGURE 26. Medical problems associated with various sports*

*Reproduced with permission from Wilmore, J.H. and J. Bergfeld. "A Comparison of Sports: Physiological and Medical Aspects," from *Sports Medicine and Physiology*, edited by R. H. Strauss, Philadelphia: W. B. Saunders, 1979

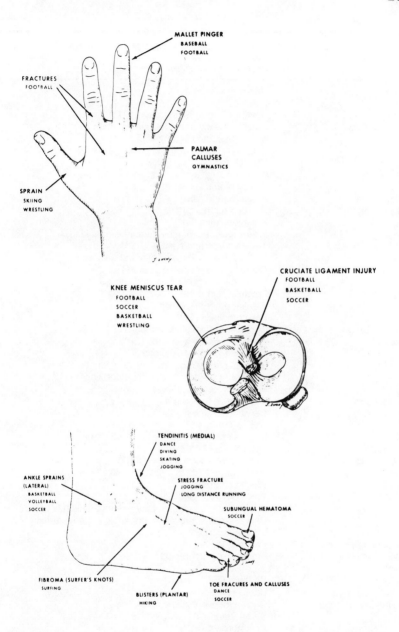

FIGURE 26. Medical problems associated with various sports (continued)

TABLE 25. Medical problems associated with various sports*

SPORT	MEDICAL PROBLEMS
Auto racing	Heat exhaustion (E)**
	Burns (E)**
	Severe life-threatening trauma (T)**
Backpacking	Brachial plexis (shoulder nerves) injury (T)**
Baseball	Mallet (baseball) finger (T)**
	Shoulder (rotator cuff) tendinitis (O)**
	Little League elbow (O)**
Basketball	Posterior tibial tendinitis at ankle (O)**
	Ankle sprains (T)**
Crew	Forearm tendinitis (O)**
Cross-Country	Stress fracture (O)**
	Knee tendinitis (O)**
Dance	Flexor halluces (big toe) tendinitis at ankle (O)**
	Toe fractures and calluses (O)**
Diving (springboard)	Cervical (neck) spine sprain and fracture (T)**
	Contusion from striking board (T)**
	Flexor halluces (big toe) tendinitis (O)**
Equestrian	Fracture of clavicle (collarbone) (T)**
	Patellar (knee) tendinitis (O)**
Fencing	Wrist tendinitis (O)**
Field Hockey	Contusions from stick and ball (T)**
Football	Bursitis at elbow and knee (E)**
	Cervical (neck) nerve pinch (T)**
	Brachial plexus (shoulder nerve) injury (T)**
	Ligament sprains at knee, shoulder, finger (T)**
	Knee meniscus (cartilage) injury (T)**
Gymnastics	Calluses on hands (O)**
Hang-Gliding	Cervical fracture (T)**
	Severe life-threatening trauma (T)**
Hiking	Blisters of the feet (O)**
Ice Hockey	Lacerations (T)**
Ice Skating	Tendinitis of foot and ankle (O)**
Javelin	Shoulder and elbow tendinitis (O)**
Jockey	Weight control (E)**
Jogging and Distance Running	Ankle and foot tendinitis (O)**
	Stress fractures of tibia, fibula, metatarsals (O)**
	Chondromalacia patellae (softening of undersurface of kneecap) (O)**
Mountain Climbing	Frostbite (E)**
Pole Vault	Fracture of humerus (O, T)**
Sailing	Seasickness (E)**
	Sunburn (E)**
	Stress reactions (peptic ulcer) (I)**
Scuba Diving	Decompression sickness (E)**
	Barotrauma (E)**
	Air embolism (E)**
Shooting (skeet)	Auditory trauma (E)**

*Reproduced with permission from, Wilmore J. H. and J. Bergfeld. A Comparison of Sports: Physiological and Medical Aspects, from *Sports Medicine and Physiology*, edited by R. H. Strauss, Philadelphia: W. B. Saunders, 1979

**The category into which each problem falls is indicated as follows: trauma (T); overuse (O); environment (E); and illness (I).

TABLE 25. Medical problems associated with various sports (continued)

SPORT	MEDICAL PROBLEMS
Shot put	Chondromalacia patellae (O, T)**
Skateboard	Contusions and abrasions of knees and elbows (T)**
Skiing (snow)	
Alpine	Tibial fractures (T)**
	Thumb sprain (T)**
Cross-Country	Frostbite (E)**
Sky Diving	Ankle fracture (T)**
Snowmobiling	Compression fracture of thoracic spine (T)**
Soccer	Hematoma under nail of big toe (T)**
	Knee meniscus and ligament injury (T)**
	Skin abrasion (E)
Sprint	Hamstring strains (O)'**
Squash	Eye injury (T)**
Surfboard	Fibroma of knee and dorsum of foot (surfer's knots) (T)**
Swimming	Eye irritation (conjunctivitis) (E)**
	Ear infection (otitis externa) (E)**
	Shoulder tendinitis (O)**
	Drowning (E)**
Tennis	Sprain of gastrocnemius (calf) muscle-tendon junction (O)**
	Tendinitis of elbow (O)**
Trampoline	Cervical (neck) spine fracture (T)**
Volleyball	Elbow and knee contusions (T)**
	Ankle sprains (T)**
Water Skiing	Knee ligament sprains (T)**
Weightlifting	Lumbar (low back) sprains (O)**
	Tendinitis (multiple locations) (O)**
Wrestling	Hematoma of ear (cauliflower ear) (T)**
	Skin infections (herpes, staphylococcal) (E)**
	Costochondral (rib) separation (T)**
	Weight control (E)**

PREVENTION OF ATHLETIC INJURIES

One of the first steps in preventing injury is to be familiar with the major types of injuries which characterize a specific sport or activity. Recognizing the potential for injury alerts the individual to be particularly sensitive to and avoid, if possible, those factors which might lead to such an injury. Ankle sprains are one of the more common medical problems in basketball. Recognizing this, many basketball teams require their athletes to tape their ankles in an attempt to provide greater stability to the joint, and to reduce the risk of serious ankle sprains. This is referred to as preventive taping.

The equipment that is used in the specific activity must be properly fitted and wisely selected. A major problem exists in the sport of football relative to the design and construction of helmets. Individual lawsuits for hundreds of thousands, and even millions, of dollars have been filed against equipment manufacturers for the faulty design of the protective headwear, which resulted in serious injury, and even death. The design and construction of the helmet may not have been the problem at all. It may have simply been a matter of a poor fit, or the alignment of the body at the time of impact. A poorly fitting shoe will cause the jogger continual problems of an annoying, and possibly incapacitating, nature—problems which could have been avoided with a proper fitting.

The environment is also a major factor associated with injuries, and can be controlled to a certain extent. The playing surface is responsible for many injuries. Holes or ruts on fields, sand on bicycle paths, and water on the basketball or tennis court are just a few of many examples of how the playing surface can contribute to the injury. A careful survey of the existing conditions prior to getting swept up in the enthusiasm of the competition can prevent serious injury. The weather conditions are also an extremely important factor which can significantly contribute to the increased risk of injury. As was discussed in Chapter 9, there are serious heat- and cold-related injuries which can be prevented by proper hydration, appropriate clothing, the scheduling of workouts or competition at a time of day when the weather conditions will be more favorable, and even canceling or postponing a workout or competition if the weather conditions exceed a certain critical level. The time of day one exercises or competes is also associated with increased or decreased risk for injury. Exercise should be avoided in the heat of the day, or at that time of day when pollution levels are at their peak. Jogging or bicycling on city streets during rush-hour traffic should also be avoided. Finally, if exercise is performed at a time when it is dark, either in the evening or early morning, precautions should be taken to assure proper lighting to avoid tripping or stumbling over an unseen object, and proper safety to reduce the chances of being mugged or assaulted.

Learning to play the game or sport properly is extremely important, which implies that the competitive rules will be followed. Rules serve various purposes, but one major purpose is to provide as safe and injury-free a situation as possible for that sport. Improper techniques are a major source of sports injuries. Poor body mechanics place the individual in a most vulnerable position for injury. Landing on the wrong part of the foot when jogging and having the head in the wrong place when making a tackle in football are examples of improper body mechanics. The appropriate strategies for a sport must be learned. Having incorrect court or field position can place the individual in a precarious position for injury. As one gains experience, he learns to avoid certain situations that have high injury potential, and he has developed a level of skill which will also provide a degree of protection. However, with experience comes repeated exposure, and with increased exposure comes an increased risk for injury.

As an example, the longer one is on a football field in the heat of battle, the greater the opportunity for injury. The third-string quarterback who never gets into the game is at a very low risk for injury.

Having an appropriate medical clearance is, in reality, the first step in an injury prevention program. Screening out those individuals who are at a significant risk for injury is important. The prospective football player with bad knees, the recreational weightlifter with high blood pressure, and the long-distance runner who is a diabetic should each receive special counsel, either encouraging them to seek another sport, or providing them with specific information that will allow them to compete at a lower risk. The medical examination should be designed for the sport. For the young football player, the examination should be heavily oriented toward the diagnosis of orthopedic problems or complications, while the examination for the middle-aged jogger should be oriented toward the diagnosis of respiratory and cardiovascular problems. For those 35 years of age and older, an exercise electrocardiogram is recommended.

Finally, being properly conditioned for the sport is probably the most important factor in injury prevention. Many injuries are the result of the individual's simply not being prepared to handle the physical stress associated with the sport. Also, as the individual begins to fatigue, he is much more susceptible to injury, for he doesn't think as clearly, or respond as quickly, move as rapidly, or hit as hard as he did when he was fresh. Being properly conditioned will not eliminate fatigue, but it will enable the individual to handle considerably more physical stress before its onset, and he will be able to function more effectively under conditions of fatigue. Appropriate levels of strength and flexibility will prevent many musculoskeletal-types of injuries, and proper cardiorespiratory and muscular endurance will reduce those problems associated with fatigue. Finally, taking the time to stretch and warm up prior to exercise and competition will prevent many injuries.

ACUTE TREATMENT OF INJURIES OR OTHER MEDICAL PROBLEMS

An injury should be treated just as soon as possible. Frequently, the length of time between the onset of injury and the initial stages of treatment can dictate the period of recovery and convalescence. For any injury of a potentially serious nature, such as head or eye injuries, fractures and chest pains, the individual and/or the specific part of the body which was injured should be immobilized. Standard first-aid procedures should be applied, and medical assistance should be obtained as quickly as possible. For injuries of a less serious nature, such as sprains, strains, and exposed wounds of a minor nature, immobilization, elevation, and ice is the usual sequence of treatments to follow. Compression of the injured area with an elastic bandage is also an effective treatment. Immobilization is necessary to prevent further damage and to reduce the pain associated with the injury. Elevation and ice are applied in an attempt to minimize and reduce swelling of or around the injured area. Once the situation has stabilized, the individual should seek medical attention. In the case of a suspected sprain, the physician may order an X ray to rule out the possibility of a fracture.

For overuse types of injuries, such as tendinitis, bursitis, shin splints, and bone bruises, frequently these will not require immediate medical attention. Rest and ice appear to be effective in the treatment of most overuse injuries; however, should the injury persist, medical consultation should be obtained. In most overuse types of injuries, the problem is compounded by the unwillingness of the individual to rest, and stay away from the stresses that caused the injury. Sometimes other activities of a less stressful nature, such as swimming and bicycling, can be substituted for the primary activity, allowing the individual to remain active while relieving the stresses associated with the primary activity. The jogger who develops a knee or ankle injury can possibly continue jogging by moving into the swimming pool in chest-deep water. The buoyancy force of the water considerably reduces the undersirable influence of gravity, and allows exercise with minimal weight-bearing. Bicycling, either stationary or free cycling, also allows vigorous exercise without the stress of weight bearing.

Various treatment modalities are available to the individual at home which do not require special equipment or preparations. Over the past 10 years, one of the biggest breakthroughs in the treatment of athletic injuries has been the development of cryokinetics, or ice therapy. The immediate application of ice to an injury is now recognized as one of the most important aspects of the total treatment program. While the direct application of ice is initially painful, or at least uncomfortable, it does eventually reduce the direct pain resulting from the injury, relaxes the underlying muscles, reduces muscle spasms, and reduces surface blood flow while increasing deep blood flow, thus reducing swelling. Icing the injury will eventually lead to numbness of the surrounding area, and the injured joint can then be passively moved without pain throughout the complete range of motion. This passive-movement treatment should be used only when the possibility of a fracture or serious sprain has been ruled out.

Heat can also be used effectively in the long-term rehabilitation of an athletic injury, but not within the first 48 to 72 hours of injury. Heat increases local circulation and allows the underlying muscles to relax. Since heat can cause additional swelling, heat treatment should not be started until there has been a reduction in the initial swelling. When heat is used, wet heat appears to have a deeper, more penetrating effect. Hot, soaked towels, hydrocollator packs, hot baths, and whirlpools are good sources of wet heat.

Massage, taping, padding, and bracing are also helpful treatment modalities, but they should be used only by an individual who is trained in the use of these modalities, such as a physical therapist or an athletic trainer. Frequently, more harm than good can result when an individual undertakes his own therapy program without appropriate advice and supervision.

At what point can the individual return to that activity in which the injury was sustained? For any serious injury, this is a decision which can be made only by the physician, therapist, or trainer who is familiar with the injury and has been involved in the rehabilitation program. It is much better to take a conservative approach at this point, for the premature return to the sport could result in a far more serious injury. For those injuries of a lesser nature, the individual should not return to the activity until the injured area is restored to its full range of motion, and until normal strength, power, and muscular endurance have been restored. The uninjured limb can be used in comparison to the injured limb to determine the extent of full recovery. Movement should be free of hitches, limping, or any other abnormal or undesirable movement patterns. Finally, movement should be pain-free. Whenever pain is still present, the individual will have a tendency to favor that area, which can create additional problems in other parts of the body.

Most of the information presented in this section has been directed toward musculoskeletal injuries. There are also problems of a cardiovascular nature which must be considered. The participant must be aware of the various warning signs that may occur during or following strenuous exercise. Dr. Lenore Zohman, a prominent cardiologist in New York City, has devoted a number of years to the study of exercise prescription for the healthy as well as for those with specific cardiovascular diseases. In her booklet, "Beyond Diet . . . Exercise Your Way to Fitness and Heart Health,"* Dr. Zohman has listed a number of potential warning signs and symptoms that could occur during or immediately following exercise. These may be grouped into the following two categories:

    A. Stop Exercising. See a physician before resuming.
        1. Abnormal heart activity, including irregular pulse (missed beats or extra beats), fluttering, jumping, or palpitations in the chest or throat, sudden burst of rapid heartbeats, or a sudden slowing of a rapid pulse rate

---

*Zohman, L. "Beyond Diet . . . Exercise Your Way to Fitness and Heart Health," Englewood Cliffs, New Jersey: Mazola Products, Best Foods, 1974. (available through the local affiliate of the American Heart Association)

2. Pain or pressure in the center of the chest, or the arm or throat, during or immediately following exercise

3. Dizziness, lightheadedness, sudden lack of coordination, confusion, cold sweating, glassy stare, pallor, blueness, or fainting

4. Illness, particularly viral infections, can lead to myocarditis, *i.e.*, viral infection of the heart muscle. Avoid exercise during and immediately following an illness.

B. Attempt Self-Correction.

1. Persistent rapid pulse rate throughout 5 to 10 minutes of recovery or longer
   Self-Correction Technique: reduce the intensity of the activity (use a lower training heart rate) and progress to higher levels of activity at a slower rate. Consult a physician if the condition persists.

2. Nausea or vomiting after exercise
   Self-Correction Technique: reduce the intensity of the endurance exercise and prolong the cool-down period. Avoid eating for at least 2 hours prior to the exercise session.

3. Extreme breathlessness lasting more than 10 minutes after the cessation of exercise
   Self-Correction Technique: reduce the intensity of the endurance exercise. Consult a physician if the condition persists.

4. Prolonged fatigue up to 24 hours following exercise
   Self-Correction Technique: reduce the intensity of the endurance exercise and reduce the duration of the total workout session if this symptom persists. Consult a physician if these self-correcting techniques do not remedy the situation.

Appendix

The Skeleton

The skeleton is comprised of two parts, the *axial skeleton* and the *appendicular skeleton*. The axial skeleton is composed of the bones of the skull, the vertebral column, and the thorax. The appendicular skeleton is composed of the bones in the upper and lower extremity. The adult skeleton consists of a total of 206 bones.

Bones have surfaces which include various projections and depressions which have important functions relative to the use of the bone. A *process* is a general term for any bony projection. A *spine* or *spinous* process is a sharp projection, while a *tubercle* and *tuberosity* are small and large rounded projections, respectively. A *trochanter* is a very large process; a *condyle* is a rounded or knuckle-like process for articulation; a *crest* is a prominent ridge; and a *head* is an enlargement at the end of the bone just beyond the constricted portion which is referred to as the neck. A *fossa* is a pit or hollow, while a *groove* and a *sulcus* are furrows. A *sinus* is a cavity, a *foramen* is a hole or opening, and a *meatus* is a tube-like passage.

Axial Skeleton. As was mentioned above, the axial skeleton is comprised of the skull (29 bones), the vertebral column (26 bones), and the thorax (25 bones). In the skull, the 8 bones of the cranium form the floor and a dome-like vault that encase the brain. Of the 14 bones that form the face, the mandible, or lower jaw bone, and the maxilla, or the upper jaw bone, and the nasal bones forming the nose are of greatest significance. An additional 6 bones are found in the 2 ears (3 bones per ear), and the last, or twenty-ninth bone, the hyoid bone, is not truly a bone of the skull, as it is located in the upper neck.

The vertebral column or spine is a series of bones or *vertebrae* that form a column which provides support for the skull, a base for the ribs, and

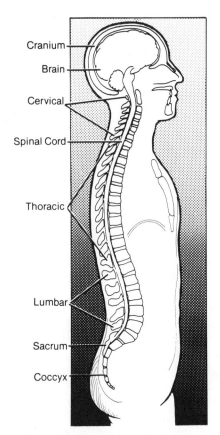

FIGURE 27. The vertebral column

encloses the spinal cord. There are a total of 33 vertebrae, which are divided into 5 groups according to their characteristics and location. Going from the head to the tail, the *cervical vertebrae* are 7 in number, and start at the base of the skull and form the neck. Next, the *thoracic vertebrae*, 12 in number, form the upper back and give rise to the 12 ribs. The *lumbar vertebrae*, 5 in number, form the lower back. The *sacrum* is formed by the fusion of 5 vertebrae and is frequently considered a single bone. Finally, the *coccyx* is comprised of 4 or 5 vertebrae which are fused into a single bone, which is also referred to as the tail bone.

The *thorax* is a large bony cage which provides structure for the chest wall. It is comprised of 24 ribs, 12 on each side of the body, and the *sternum,* or breast bone. Each rib is attached to one of the thoracic vertebrae in the back, and to the sternum or cartilage in the front, with the exception of the bottom two, or the eleventh and twelfth ribs, which have no attachment on the front side of the body, and are thus referred to as floating ribs. The sternum has three parts: the upper part, or manubrium; the middle part, or body; and the lower part, or the xiphoid process.

Appendicular Skeleton. The upper and lower extremities comprise the appendicular skeleton. The upper extremity is composed of the shoulder, including the *scapula* and the *clavicle,* the upper arm, forearm, wrist, and hand. The scapula is a triangle-shaped bone located in the upper back region, and is frequently referred to as the shoulder blade. The clavicle is a slender bone that separates the sternum from the shoulder joint, providing support for the shoulder joint. The bone of the upper arm is the *humerus,* while the forearm is composed of 2 bones, the *radius* and the *ulna.* The wrist is comprised of 8 small bones referred to as *carpal bones,* while the hand is comprised of 5 *metacarpals* and 14 *phalanges.* The metacarpals form the palm of the hand and the phalanges form the fingers, 3 phalanges per finger and 2 for the thumb.

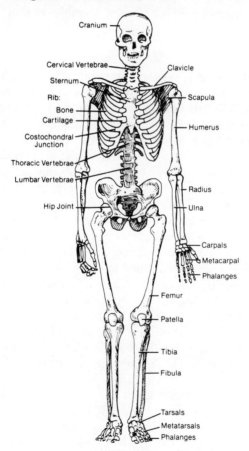

FIGURE 28. The human skeleton

The lower extremity is comprised of the hip or pelvic girdle, the upper and lower legs, the kneecap and the foot, including the ankle. The pelvic girdle serves to unite the vertebral column with the lower body, and provides a rather wide basin of support and protection for many of the body organs. The bone of the upper leg is the massive *femur,* which is the longest and strongest bone in the body. The kneecap, or *patella,* is a rather small oval-shaped bone which covers and protects the knee joint, and provides a point of attachment for muscles, which increases their leverage. The lower leg is formed by the large and thick *tibia* which lies on the inside of the leg, and the smaller and thinner *fibula* which lies on the outside. The front edge of the tibia commonly is referred to as the shin bone. The ankle is comprised of 7 bones referred to as *tarsal bones.* The foot is composed of 5 *metatarsal* bones, and the toes include 14 *phalanges,* 2 for the big toe and 3 each for the remaining toes. In many respects, the structure of the foot closely resembles that of the hand.

Articulations

The bones of the skeletal system join together to form the supporting framework of the body. Whenever 2 or more bones meet, articulations or joints are formed. The articulation of the femur with the tibia forms the knee joint. The humerus articulates with the radius and ulna to form the elbow joint. And the 3 phalanges of each finger articulate to form several joints for each finger. Several types of joints exist in the body. Essentially there are 3 primary classifications of joints: fibrous, cartilaginous, and synovial. *Fibrous joints* are those joints where bones are essentially joined together by fibrous-like elastic connective tissue, allowing little or no movement. The bones of the cranium or skullcap are joined together in this fashion. *Cartilaginous joints* are similar in characteristic, there being no space or joint cavity between bones, and there is only limited motion. The bodies of the vertebrae are joined in this manner. *Synovial joints* are of the greatest importance for purposes of discussion in this book. Synovial joints are formed by the articulating bones, a thin layer of cartilage on the ends of the bones and a fibrous capsule that encloses the joint. All the joints of the extremities are synovial joints. The fibrous joint capsule is lined on the inside with a membrane which has a rich capillary network of blood vessels. This membrane is referred to as the *synovial membrane,* and it produces a viscous or relatively thick fluid, *synovial fluid,* which provides a natural lubrication for all joint movement. The smooth hyaline cartilage on the ends of those bones involved in the articulation provides a surface which has a greatly reduced friction, and which when combined with the synovial fluid provides a relatively free motion within the joint.

A disc of fibrous cartilage is present in some joints, dividing the joint cavity and providing a smoother surface for joint action. The knee joint has several of these discs, or menisci, which allow for a better articulation of the femur with the tibia. Frequently, when the knee is injured in athletics, the meniscus is damaged and must be removed through surgery. However, loss of one or both menisci in a single knee joint does not greatly limit joint movement, although the articulation is not as smooth and joint swelling and pain are often the result, with the possibility of arthritis in the later years.

Ligaments are cords or bands of fibrous tissue which cross the joint, attaching one bone to another, providing strength to the joint capsule, so it won't be pulled apart or disrupted in any fashion. Ligaments typically lie outside the joint capsule, but are also found within the joint capsule for certain joints, *e.g.*, cruciate ligaments inside the knee joint. *Tendons* are formed of connective tissue and provide the means by which muscles are attached to bones. Tendons cross joints and, thus, provide additional support for that specific joint. *Bursae* are small sacs that are filled with synovial fluid and are present in the area of joints where tendons are likely to rub against bone, against ligaments or against other tendons, or at locations where skin moves over a bony prominence. They function to reduce friction at these points of movement.

Joints can move in any one of a number of different ways. *Flexion* and *extension* are movements where the angle between the bones forming the joints decreases and increases, respectively. As an example, in the elbow joint, flexion occurs as the forearm is closing on the upper arm, decreasing the joint angle, such as when one flexes his arm to accentuate the size of the biceps muscle. Extension occurs when the forearm is straightened out, increasing the joint angle. Extension and flexion of the foot have a special terminology. Foot flexion, bringing the toes toward the lower leg, is referred to as *dorsi-flexion,* while foot extension is referred to as *plantar-flexion,* plantar having reference to the bottom of the foot. *Abduction* refers to movement away from the midline of the body toward the side, such as raising the arm at the shoulder joint to the side. *Adduction* refers to movement toward the midline of the body, such as lowering the arm at the shoulder joint back to the side of the body. *Circumduction* is movement in a circular motion, such as making a circling movement with the arm at the shoulder joint. *Rotation* is movement around an axis. Several types of rotation have specific terms. *Supination* involves turning the palm of the hand and the forearm upward, and *pronation* involves turning the palm of the hand and the forearm downward. Rotation of the bottom or plantar surface of the foot outward is referred to as *eversion,* and rotation of the bottom surface of the foot inward is referred to as *inversion.*

Skeletal Muscles of the Human Body

The human body has a total of more than 400 muscles that act through the system of levers provided by the skeletal system to produce movement. It is not possible to describe and discuss each of these in this book, but the more important muscles, including their location and their functions, will be presented. The major muscles involved with each of the more important joints will be illustrated, and then origins, insertions, and functions will be described. A muscle's *origin* is the more fixed or less movable attachment of a muscle and serves as the base or origin of action. The muscle's *insertion* is the attachment at the more movable end of the muscle. With most limb muscles, the origins are more proximal and the insertions are more distal on the length of the bone.

The major muscles in the body are illustrated in Figures 29 through 36 (pages 229-232). Only the major muscles will be discussed due to the rather general nature of this book. Those who would like more detail should consult a current textbook of anatomy. To facilitate the presentation of rather complex information, the specific muscles to be reviewed in this book will be presented in outline form, with a description of their origin, insertion, and action or function. The muscles will be listed according to their major area of function. In some cases a muscle crosses more than one joint and has specific functions at several joints. These muscles will be listed under those areas where they exhibit their major function.

A. Muscles of the Head and Neck
    1. Sternocleidomastoid
        a. *Origin:* sternum and clavicle   *Insertion:* temporal bone
        b. *Function:* both sides acting together flex the head, acting separately bends head to the side of the contracting muscle
    2. Prevertebral muscles (deep anterior muscles of the head and neck, including longus capitis, longus colli, rectus capitus anterior and rectus capitus lateralis)
        a. *Origin:* cervical and upper   *Insertion:* occipital bone and
            three thoracic vertebrae   cervical vertebrae
        b. *Function:* both sides acting together flex head and neck, acting separately bends head to the side of the contracting muscle

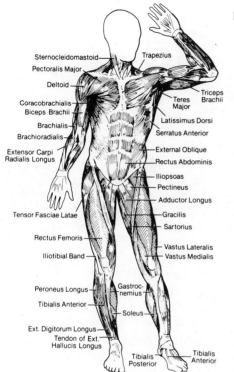

FIGURE 29. Muscles of the body viewed from the front

Sternocleidomastoid
Pectoralis Major
Deltoid
Coracobrachialis
Biceps Brachii
Brachialis
Brachioradialis
Extensor Carpi Radialis Longus
Tensor Fasciae Latae
Rectus Femoris
Iliotibial Band
Peroneus Longus
Tibialis Anterior
Ext. Digitorum Longus
Tendon of Ext. Hallucis Longus
Tibialis Posterior

Trapezius
Triceps Brachii
Teres Major
Latissimus Dorsi
Serratus Anterior
External Oblique
Rectus Abdominis
Iliopsoas
Pectineus
Adductor Longus
Gracilis
Sartorius
Vastus Lateralis
Vastus Medialis
Gastrocnemius
Soleus
Tibialis Anterior

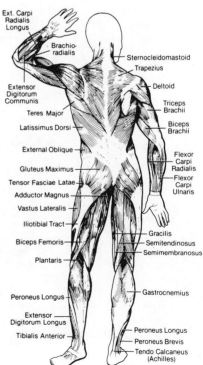

Ext. Carpi Radialis Longus
Brachioradialis
Extensor Digitorum Communis
Teres Major
Latissimus Dorsi
External Oblique
Gluteus Maximus
Tensor Fasciae Latae
Adductor Magnus
Vastus Lateralis
Iliotibial Tract
Biceps Femoris
Plantaris
Peroneus Longus
Extensor Digitorum Longus
Tibialis Anterior

Sternocleidomastoid
Trapezius
Deltoid
Triceps Brachii
Biceps Brachii
Flexor Carpi Radialis
Flexor Carpi Ulnaris
Gracilis
Semitendinosus
Semimembranosus
Gastrocnemius
Peroneus Longus
Peroneus Brevis
Tendo Calcaneus (Achilles)

FIGURE 30. Muscles of the body viewed from the rear

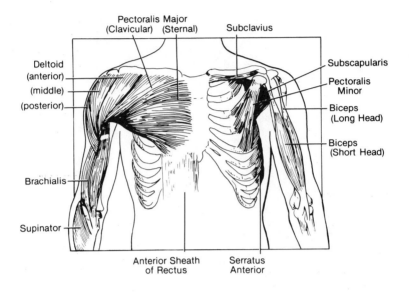

FIGURE 31. Muscles of the chest, shoulder, and arm

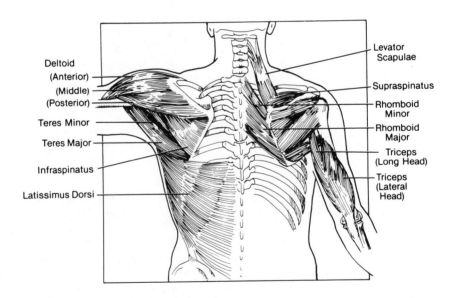

FIGURE 32. Muscles of the back, shoulder, and arm

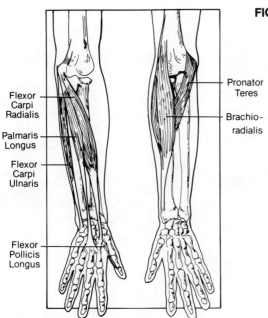

Flexor
Carpi
Radialis

Palmaris
Longus

Flexor
Carpi
Ulnaris

Flexor
Pollicis
Longus

Pronator
Teres

Brachio-
radialis

**FIGURE 33. Front view of the
muscles of the
arm and forearm**

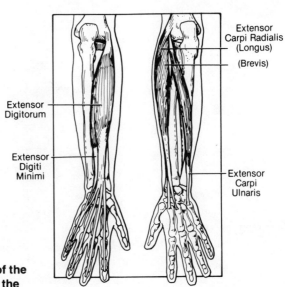

Extensor
Digitorum

Extensor
Digiti
Minimi

Extensor
Carpi Radialis
(Longus)

(Brevis)

Extensor
Carpi
Ulnaris

**FIGURE 34. Rear view of the
muscles of the
forearm**

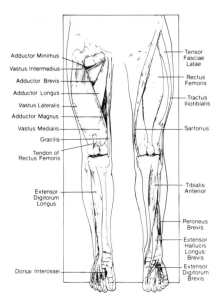

FIGURE 35. Front view of the deep and superficial muscles of the lower extremity

Adductor Minimus

Vastus Intermedius

Adductor Brevis

Adductor Longus

Vastus Lateralis

Adductor Magnus

Vastus Medialis

Gracilis

Tendon of Rectus Femoris

Extensor Digitorum Longus

Dorsal Interossei

Tensor Fasciae Latae

Rectus Femoris

Tractus Iliotibialis

Sartorius

Tibialis Anterior

Peroneus Brevis

Extensor Hallucis Longus: Brevis

Extensor Digitorum Brevis

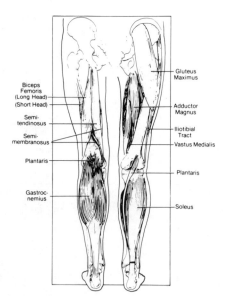

Biceps Femoris (Long Head) (Short Head)

Semi-tendinosus

Semi-membranosus

Plantaris

Gastroc-nemius

Gluteus Maximus

Adductor Magnus

Iliotibial Tract

Vastus Medialis

Plantaris

Soleus

FIGURE 36. Rear view of the deep and superficial muscles of the lower extremity

3. Hyoid muscles (including the suprahyoids and the infrahyoids)
   a. *Origin:* temporal bone and   *Insertion:* hyoid bone
     mandible above and sternum
     and scapula below
   b. *Function:* flexion of the neck
4. Scaleni muscles (anterior, posterior, and medius)
   a. *Origin:* cervical vertebrae   *Insertion:* first two ribs
   b. *Function:* both sides acting together assist in flexing the neck, acting separately bends head to the side of the contracting muscle
5. Splenius capitis and cervicis
   a. *Origin:* ligamentum nuchae   *Insertion:* temporal bone,
     and seventh cervical and first   occipital bone, and upper
     six thoracic vertebrae   three cervical vertebrae
   b. *Function:* both sides acting together extend and hyperextend the neck, acting separately bends head to the side of the contracting muscle or rotates the head to the same side
6. Suboccipitals
   a. *Origin:* first two cervical   *Insertion:* occipital bone and
     vertebrae   first cervical vertebrae
   b. *Function:* same as splenius capitis and cervicis

B. Muscles of the Vertebral Column
1. Erector spinae (3 branches: iliocostalis, longissimus, and spinalis)
   a. *Origin:* iliac crest, sacrum,   *Insertion:* thoracic vertebrae
     lumbar, and lower two   and ribs
     thoracic vertebrae
   b. *Function:* extension of vertebral column
2. Semispinalis (thoracis, cervicis, and capitis)
   a. *Origin:* thoracic and lower   *Insertion:* upper five thoracic
     four cervical vertebrae   and cervical vertebrae, and
         the occipital bone
   b. *Function:* extension, hyperextension and rotation of head, neck, and upper vertebral column
3. Deep posterior muscles of the spine (multifidus, rotatores, interspinalis, intertransversarii, and levatores costarum)
   a. *Origin:* sacrum and vertebrae   *Insertion:* vertebrae above
   b. *Function:* both sides acting together extend and hyperextend the vertebral column, acting separately rotate to the opposite side and assist in bending to the same side

C. Muscles of the Abdomen
   1. Rectus abdominus
      a. *Origin:* crest of the pubis   *Insertion:* fifth, sixth, and
                                           seventh ribs, and sternum
      b. *Function:* both sides acting together flex the vertebral column,
         acting separately lateral flexion to the same side as
         the contracting muscle
   2. External abdominal oblique
      a. *Origin:* lower eight ribs   *Insertion:* iliac crest and
                                         aponeurosis from ribs to
                                         pubic crest
      b. *Function:* both sides acting together flex the vertebral column,
         acting separately lateral flexion to the same side as
         the contracting muscle and rotation to the opposite
         side
   3. Internal abdominal oblique
      a. *Origin:* inguinal ligament and   *Insertion:* lower three ribs
         iliac crest   and sternum
      b. *Function:* both sides acting together flex the vertebral column,
         acting separately lateral flexion and rotation to the
         same side as the contracting muscle
   4. Transverse abdominus
      a. *Origin:* inguinal ligament,   *Insertion:* sternum, linea
         iliac crest, and lower six ribs   alba, and pubic crest
      b. *Function:* constriction of abdomen
   5. Quadratus lumborum
      a. *Origin:* iliac crest   *Insertion:* twelfth rib and
                                    upper four lumbar vertebrae
      b. *Function:* both sides acting together stabilize the pelvis and
         lumbar spine, acting separately flexes lumbar spine
         to the same side
D. Muscles of the Shoulder Joint and Shoulder Girdle
   1. Subclavius
      a. *Origin:* first rib   *Insertion:* clavicle
      b. *Function:* depression of clavicle and stabilization of sterno-
         clavicular joint.
   2. Pectoralis Minor
      a. *Origin:* third, fourth, and   *Insertion:* scapula
         fifth ribs
      b. *Function:* downward rotation of scapula and depression of
         shoulder
   3. Pectoralis Major
      a. *Origin:* clavicle, sternum, and   *Insertion:* humerus, just
         first six ribs   below the head
      b. *Function:* flexion, adduction and medial rotation of the arm

4. Serratus anterior
   a. *Origin:* upper nine ribs   *Insertion:* vertebral border and inferior angle of the scapula
   b. *Function:* abduction of vertebral border of the scapula and rotation of the scapula
5. Levator scapula
   a. *Origin:* first four cervical vertebrae   *Insertion:* vertebral border of the scapula
   b. *Function:* elevation of the scapula, slight rotation of the scapula
6. Trapezius
   a. *Origin:* occipital bone, ligamentum nuchae, and seventh cervical and all thoracic vertebrae   *Insertion:* clavicle and scapula
   b. *Function:* elevation, adduction, upward rotation, and depression of the scapula
7. Rhomboids (major and minor)
   a. *Origin:* ligamentum nuchae, seventh cervical, and first five thoracic vertebrae   *Insertion:* vertebral border of the scapula
   b. *Function:* downward rotation, adduction, and elevation of the scapula
8. Deltoid
   a. *Origin:* clavicle and scapula   *Insertion:* humerus
   b. *Function:* abduction of arm; flexion, extension, and rotation of arm when separate parts of the deltoid contract
9. Supraspinatus
   a. *Origin:* scapula   *Insertion:* humerus
   b. *Function:* abduction of the arm
10. Infraspinatus and teres minor
    a. *Origin:* scapula   *Insertion:* humerus
    b. *Function:* outward rotation and adduction of the arm
11. Teres major
    a. *Origin:* scapula   *Insertion:* humerus
    b. *Function:* adduction, extension, and inward rotation of the arm
12. Subscapularis
    a. *Origin:* scapula   *Insertion:* humerus
    b. *Function:* inward rotation of the arm, and aids in adduction, abduction, flexion, and extension of the arm

13. Coracobrachialis
   a. *Origin:* scapula   *Insertion:* humerus
   b. *Function:* flexion and adduction of the arm
14. Latissimus dorsi
   a. *Origin:* lower six thoracic   *Insertion:* humerus
      and all lumbar vertebrae,
      sacrum, iliac crest, and lower
      three ribs
   b. *Function:* adduction, extension and inward rotation of the
      arm, and draws shoulder backward and downward
E. Muscles of the Arm and Forearm
   1. Biceps brachii
      a. *Origin:* scapula   *Insertion:* radius
      b. *Function:* flexion of the arm and forearm, and supination of
         hand
   2. Brachialis
      a. *Origin:* humerus   *Insertion:* ulna
      b. *Function:* flexion of the forearm
   3. Brachioradialis
      a. *Origin:* humerus   *Insertion:* radius
      b. *Function:* flexion of the forearm
   4. Triceps brachii
      a. *Origin:* scapula and humerus   *Insertion:* ulna
      b. *Function:* extension of the forearm
   5. Pronator quadratus
      a. *Origin:* ulna   *Insertion:* radius
      b. *Function:* pronation of forearm
   6. Pronator teres
      a. *Origin:* humerus and ulna   *Insertion:* radius
      b. *Function:* pronation of forearm and assists in flexion of the
         forearm
   7. Anconeus
      a. *Origin:* humerus   *Insertion:* ulna
      b. *Function:* extension of the forearm
   8. Supinator
      a. *Origin:* humerus and ulna   *Insertion:* radius
      b. *Function:* supination of the forearm
   9. Palmaris longus
      a. *Origin:* humerus   *Insertion:* transverse carpal
         ligament and palmar
         asponeurosis
      b. *Function:* flexion of the wrist and forearm

10. Flexor carpi radialis
    a. *Origin:* humerus   *Insertion:* second metacarpal
    b. *Function:* flexion and abduction of the wrist and assists in flexion of the forearm
11. Flexor carpi ulnaris
    a. *Origin:* humerus and ulna   *Insertion:* carpal bones and fifth metacarpal
    b. *Function:* flexion and adduction of the wrist and assists in flexion of the forearm
12. Extensor carpi radialis longus
    a. *Origin:* humerus   *Insertion:* second metacarpal
    b. *Function:* extension and abduction of the wrist
13. Extensor carpi radialis brevis
    a. *Origin:* humerus   *Insertion:* third metacarpal
    b. *Function:* extension and abduction of the wrist, and assists in flexion of the forearm
14. Extensor carpi ulnaris
    a. *Origin:* humerus and ulna   *Insertion:* base of fifth metacarpal
    b. *Function:* extension and adduction of the wrist, and assists in flexion of the forearm
15. Flexor digitorum superficialis
    a. *Origin:* humerus, ulna, and radius   *Insertion:* middle phalanx of the four fingers
    b. *Function:* flexion of the fingers and wrist
16. Flexor digitorum profundus
    a. *Origin:* ulna   *Insertion:* distal phalanx of the four fingers
    b. *Function:* flexion of the fingers and wrist
17. Flexor pollicis longus
    a. *Origin:* radius and ulna   *Insertion:* distal phalanx of thumb
    b. *Function:* flexion of the thumb and wrist
18. Extensor digitorum
    a. *Origin:* humerus   *Insertion:* middle and distal phalanx of the four fingers
    b. *Function:* extension of the fingers and wrist
19. Extensor indicis
    a. *Origin:* ulna   *Insertion:* index finger
    b. *Function:* extension of index finger and assists in the extension of the wrist

20. Extensor digiti minimi
    a. *Origin:* humerus and   *Insertion:* little finger
       proximal tendon of extensor
       digitorum
    b. *Function:* extension of the little finger and assists in the exten-
       sion of the wrist
21. Extensor pollicis longus
    a. *Origin:* ulna   *Insertion:* distal phalanx of
       the thumb
    b. *Function:* extension of the thumb, and assists in the flexion
       and abduction of the wrist
22. Extensor pollicis brevis
    a. *Origin:* radius   *Insertion:* first phalanx of
       thumb
    b. *Function:* extension of the thumb
23. Abductor pollicis longus
    a. *Origin:* ulna and radius   *Insertion:* base of first
       metacarpal
    b. *Function:* extension and abduction of the thumb

F. Muscles of the Hip
    1. Psoas (major and minor)
       a. *Origin:* twelfth thoracic and   *Insertion:* femur
          all lumbar vertebrae
       b. *Function:* flexion of pelvis on abdomen, flexion and medial
          rotation of the thigh, and flexion of lumbar region of
          vertebral column
    2. Iliacus
       a. *Origin:* ilium and sacrum   *Insertion:* femur
       b. *Function:* flexion and lateral rotation of the thigh
    3. Gluteus maximus
       a. *Origin:* ilium, sacrum, and   *Insertion:* femur
          coccyx
       b. *Function:* extension and lateral rotation of the thigh
    4. Gluteus medius and minimus
       a. *Origin:* ilium   *Insertion:* femur
       b. *Function:* abduction and medial rotation of the thigh
    5. Tensor fasciae latae
       a. *Origin:* iliac crest and iliac   *Insertion:* femur
          spine
       b. *Function:* flexion, medial rotation, and abduction of the thigh
    6. Six deep lateral rotators (obturator externus and internus, gemel-
       lus superior and inferior, quadratus femoris, and piriformis)
       a. *Origin:* sacrum and pelvis   *Insertion:* femur
       b. *Function:* lateral rotation of the thigh

7. Pectineus
   a. *Origin:* pubis   *Insertion:* femur
   b. *Function:* flexion, adduction, and lateral rotation of the thigh
G. Muscles of the Thigh
   1. Sartorius
      a. *Origin:* iliac spine   *Insertion:* tibia
      b. *Function:* flexion and lateral rotation of the thigh, flexion and medial rotation of the leg
   2. Quadriceps femoris (rectus femoris, and vastus lateralis, medialis and intermedius)
      a. *Origin:* pelvis and femur   *Insertion:* patella
      b. *Function:* flexion of the thigh (rectus femoris) and extension of the leg
   3. Gracilis
      a. *Origin:* pubis   *Insertion:* tibia
      b. *Function:* adduction of the thigh and flexion of the leg
   4. Adductors (longus, magnus, and brevis)
      a. *Origin:* pubis and ischium   *Insertion:* femur
      b. *Function:* adduction, flexion (longus and brevis), extension (magnus), and lateral rotation of the thigh
   5. Biceps femoris
      a. *Origin:* ischium and femur   *Insertion:* fibula and tibia
      b. *Function:* extension of the thigh, and flexion and lateral rotation of the leg
   6. Semitendinosus
      a. *Origin:* ischium   *Insertion:* tibia
      b. *Function:* extension of the thigh, and flexion and medial rotation of the leg
   7. Semimembranosus
      a. *Origin:* ischium   *Insertion:* tibia
      b. *Function:* extension of the thigh, and flexion and medial rotation of the leg
H. Muscles of the Leg
   1. Tibialis anterior
      a. *Origin:* tibia   *Insertion:* first metatarsal and first cuneiform
      b. *Function:* dorsal flexion and supination of the foot
   2. Extensor digitorum longus
      a. *Origin:* tibia and fibula   *Insertion:* second and third phalanges of the four lesser toes
      b. *Function:* dorsal flexion and pronation of the foot, and extension of the toes

3. Extensor hallucis longus
   a. *Origin:* fibula   *Insertion:* distal phalanx of big toe
   b. *Function:* dorsal flexion and eversion of the foot, and extension of big toe
4. Peroneus tertius
   a. *Origin:* fibula   *Insertion:* base of fifth metatarsal
   b. *Function:* dorsal flexion and pronation of the foot
5. Peroneus brevis
   a. *Origin:* fibula   *Insertion:* base of fifth metatarsal
   b. *Function:* plantar flexion and pronation of the foot
6. Peroneus longus
   a. *Origin:* tibia and fibula   *Insertion:* first cuneiform and base of first metatarsal
   b. *Function:* plantar flexion and pronation of the foot
7. Gastrocnemius
   a. *Origin:* femur   *Insertion:* calcaneus bone of the foot
   b. *Function:* plantar flexion of the foot and flexion of the leg
8. Soleus
   a. *Origin:* fibula and tibia   *Insertion:* calcaneus bone of the foot
   b. *Function:* plantar flexion of the foot
9. Tibialis posterior
   a. *Origin:* tibia and fibula   *Insertion:* navicular and calcaneus bones of the foot, three cuneiforms, cuboid bone, and bases of second to fourth metatarsals
   b. *Function:* plantar flexion and supination of the foot
10. Plantaris
    a. *Origin:* femur   *Insertion:* calcaneus bone of the foot
    b. *Function:* plantar flexion of the foot and flexion of the leg
11. Popliteus
    a. *Origin:* femur   *Insertion:* tibia
    b. *Function:* flexion and medial rotation of the leg
12. Flexor digitorum longus
    a. *Origin:* tibia   *Insertion:* base of distal phalanx of the four lesser toes
    b. *Function:* flexion of the toes and plantar flexion and supination of the foot

13. Flexor hallucis longus
    a. *Origin:* fibula   *Insertion:* distal phalanx of
                  big toe
    b. *Function:* flexion of the big toe, and flexion and supination
       of the foot

Selected Readings

SECTION A.
Optimal Health Through Physical Activity and Sport

Amsterdam, E. A., J. H. Wilmore, and A. N. DeMaria, editors. *Exercise in Cardiovascular Health and Disease*. New York: Yorke Medical Books, 1977.

Fletcher, G. F. and J. D. Cantwell. *Exercise and Coronary Heart Disease*. Springfield, Illinois: Charles C Thomas, 1974.

Kraus, H. and W. Raab. *Hypokinetic Disease*. Springfield, Illinois: Charles C Thomas, 1961.

Larsen, O. A. and R. O. Malmborg, editors. *Coronary Heart Disease and Physical Fitness*. Baltimore: University Park Press, 1971.

Mayer, J. *Overweight: Causes, Cost, and Control*. Englewood Cliffs, New Jersey, 1968.

Naughton, J. P. and H. K. Hellerstein, editors. *Exercise Testing and Exercise Training in Coronary Heart Disease*. New York: Academic Press, 1973.

Pařízková, J. *Body Fat and Physical Fitness*. The Hague: Martinus Nijhoff, 1977.

Pollock, M. L., J. H. Wilmore, and S. M. Fox, III. *Health and Fitness Through Physical Activity*. New York: John Wiley & Sons, 1978.

Sonnenblick, E. H. and M. Lesch, editors. *Exercise and Heart Disease*. New York: Grune & Stratton, 1977.

Wenger, N. K., editor. *Exercise and the Heart*. Philadelphia: F. A. Davis, 1978.

Wilson, N. L., editor. *Obesity*. Philadelphia: F. A. Davis, 1969.

Winick, M., editor. *Childhood Obesity*. New York: John Wiley & Sons, 1975.

SECTION B.
The Prescription of Exercise for Fitness and Sport

Cooper, K. H. *Aerobics*. New York: M. Evans & Co., 1968.

———. *The New Aerobics*. New York: M. Evans & Co., 1970.

———. *The Aerobics Way*. New York: M. Evans & Co., 1977.

Costill, D. L. "A Scientific Approach to Distance Running." Los Altos, California: *Track and Field News*, 1979.

Daniels, J., R. Fitts, and G. Sheehan. *Conditioning for Distance Running*. New York: John Wiley & Sons, 1978.

Fahey, T. D. *The Good-Time Fitness Book*. New York: Butterick Publishing, 1978.

Faria, I. E. and P. R. Cavanagh. *The Physiology and Biomechanics of Cycling*. New York: John Wiley & Sons, 1978.

Fixx, J. F. *The Complete Book of Running*. New York: Random House, 1977.

Foss, M. L. and J. G. Garrick. *Ski Conditioning*. New York: John Wiley & Sons, 1978.

Fox, E. L. and D. K. Mathews. *Interval Training: Conditioning for Sports and General Fitness*. Philadelphia: W. B. Saunders Company, 1974.

Getchell, B. *Physical Fitness: A Way of Life*. Second edition. New York: John Wiley & Sons, 1979.

Jensen, C. R. and A. G. Fisher. *Scientific Basis of Athletic Conditioning*. Second edition. Philadelphia: Lea & Febiger, 1979.

Kuntzleman, C. T. *Activetics*. New York: Peter H. Wyden/Publisher, 1975.

O'Shea, J. P. *Scientific Principles and Methods of Strength Fitness*. Second edition. Menlo Park, California: Addison-Wesley Publishing Company, 1976.

Pollock, M. L., J. H. Wilmore, and S. M. Fox, III. *Health and Fitness Through Physical Activity*. New York: John Wiley & Sons, 1978.

Sharkey, B. J. *Physiology of Fitness*. Champaign, Illinois: Human Kinetics Publishers, 1979.

Stone, W. J. and W. A. Kroll. *Sports Conditioning and Weight Training*. Boston: Allyn and Bacon, 1978.

SECTION C.
Special Considerations Related to Exercise and Sport

Albinson, J. G. and G. M. Andrew. *Child in Sport and Physical Activity*. Baltimore: University Park Press, 1976.

American Association for Health, Physical Education, and Recreation. *Nutrition for Athletes*. Washington, D.C., 1971.

Cooper, M. and K. H. Cooper. *Aerobics for Women*. M. Evans & Co., 1972.

Fahey, T. D. *What To Do About Athletic Injuries*. New York: Butterick Publishing, 1979.

Katch, F. I. and W. D. McArdle. *Nutrition, Weight Control, and Exercise*. Boston: Houghton Mifflin Company, 1977.

Klafs, C. E. and D. D. Arnheim. *Modern Principles of Athletic Training*. Second edition. St. Louis: C. V. Mosby Company, 1969.

Klafs, C. E. and M. J. Lyon. *The Female Athlete*. St. Louis: C. V. Mosby Company, 1973.

Miller, D. M. *Coaching the Female Athlete*. Philadelphia: Lea & Febiger, 1974.

Smith, N. J. *Food for Sport*. Palo Alto, California: Bull Publishing Company, 1976.

Smith, N. J., B. Ogilvie, W. Haskell, and B. Gaillard. *Handbook for the Young Athlete*. Palo Alto, California: Bull Publishing Company, 1978.

Williams, M. H. *Nutritional Aspects of Human Physical and Athletic Performance*. Springfield, Illinois: Charles C Thomas, 1976.

Young, D. R. *Physical Performance, Fitness and Diet*. Springfield, Illinois: Charles C Thomas, 1977.

Index